ADVANCE PRAISE FOR
DANGEROUS BOOBIES

"It takes a special kind of person to turn a double mastectomy into comedy, and Caitlin Brodnick is just that kind of person: a hilariously upbeat woman who happens to have been diagnosed with the BRCA gene, a diagnosis she was determined to beat."

—Cindi Leive, editor in chief of *Glamour* magazine

"Caitlin Brodnick is fabulous. She's a survivor. And I believe she thrives in part because of her humor, warmth, and generosity of spirit. She's a funny, smart writer and she'll teach you, make you laugh, and maybe make you cry. For a minute. And then you'll laugh again."

—Sara Benincasa, author of *Real Artists Have Day Jobs* and *Agorafabulous!*

"Caitlin is smart and funny and THE person to bring a fresh, needed voice to a heavy, scary, and ubiquitous topic. She is the Breast Cancer Comedy Ambassador. This book is important."

—Ilana Glazer, comedian and co-creator of Comedy Central's *Broad City*

"Caitlin and her voice are a breath of fresh air in the cynical, snarky world we can sometimes live in. I'm constantly astounded by her ability to turn life's more difficult experiences into hilarious and inspiring reflections that make you want to live more in the moment."

> —Abbi Jacobson, comedian, author, and co-creator of Comedy Central's *Broad City*

"A refreshingly hilarious, laugh-out-loud, bestie been-there-done-that road map for surviving the precarious journey cancer inevitably throws at you."

> —Emme, model, fashion icon, public speaker, and author of *Chicken Soup for the Soul: Curvy & Confident*

"Caitlin Brodnick is a fearlessly hilarious storyteller who can find humor in the darkest scenarios. I can't wait for the masses to be exposed to her talent and wit."

> —Margot Leitman, author of *Gawky* and *Long Story Short*

"Caitlin Brodnick is a charming storyteller, an exceptional writer, and—most important—a survivor. . . . Surgery stories have never been so much fun!"

> —Selena Coppock, author of *The New Rules for Blondes*

DANGEROUS BOOBIES

Breaking Up with My Time-Bomb Breasts

CAITLIN BRODNICK

SEAL PRESS

Author's note: I have tried to re-create events and conversations from my memories of them. In order to maintain anonymity, in some instances I have changed the names and identifying characteristics of individuals and places.

Copyright © 2017 Caitlin Brodnick

Photo credits: photos on pp. 12–13 © Leslie Hassler; photos on pp. 230 and 232 © Alex Schafer

Hachette Book Group supports the right to free expression and the value of copyright. The purpose of copyright is to encourage writers and artists to produce the creative works that enrich our culture.

The scanning, uploading, and distribution of this book without permission is a theft of the author's intellectual property. If you would like permission to use material from the book (other than for review purposes), please contact permissions@hbgusa.com. Thank you for your support of the author's rights.

Seal Press
Hachette Book Group
1290 Avenue of the Americas, New York, NY 10104

Printed in the United States of America
First Edition: September 2017

Published by Seal Press, an imprint of Perseus Books, LLC, a subsidiary of Hachette Book Group, Inc.

The Hachette Speakers Bureau provides a wide range of authors for speaking events. To find out more, go to www.hachettespeakersbureau.com or call (866) 376-6591.

The publisher is not responsible for websites (or their content) that are not owned by the publisher.

Print book interior design by Amy Quinn

Library of Congress Cataloging-in-Publication Data

Names: Brodnick, Caitlin, author.
Title: Dangerous boobies : breaking up with my time-bomb breasts / Caitlin Brodnick.
Description: Berkeley, California : Seal Press, [2017]
Identifiers: LCCN 2017014654| ISBN 9781580056755 (paperback) | ISBN 9781580056762 (ebook)
Subjects: LCSH: Brodnick, Caitlin,—Health. | Breast—Cancer—Patients—New York (State)—Biography. | Mastectomy—Patients—New York (State)—Biography. | BRCA genes. | BISAC: BIOGRAPHY & AUTOBIOGRAPHY / Personal Memoirs. | HEALTH & FITNESS / Diseases / Cancer.
Classification: LCC RC280.B8 B7447 2017 | DDC 616.99/449059—dc23
LC record available at https://lccn.loc.gov/2017014654

ISBNs: 978-1-58005-675-5 (paperback), 978-1-58005-676-2 (ebook)

LSC-C

10 9 8 7 6 5 4 3 2 1

To my Bubby and my Allen

CONTENTS

FOREWORD BY RACHEL BLOOM

Every woman I have ever known has a complicated relationship with her boobs. I wouldn't call it a love/hate relationship; it's more of a hmm/ugh/what?/yeah baby!/eh relationship.

The women I know with smaller boobs are insecure about their size but are also grateful that modern fashion is made for their body type. The women I know with larger boobs are insecure about their size but are also grateful that vintage fashion is made for their body type. Women with boobs of all sizes deal with hormone-related pain, unwanted attention from men on the street, cleavage sweat pimples, breast-milk leakage, and more. Trans women deal with these problems plus the fact that many won't develop naturally fully developed breasts; trans men must shed their boobs to realize their gender identities. Even cis-gender men worry about having "man boobs" or, in rare cases, male breast cancer (yes, it happens).

Though I sometimes long for the kindergarten days when I could run around shirtless on a hot day, I am, for the most part, grateful for my boobs. Even as five-year-old me ran topless through a sprinkler, I daydreamed about someday having massive boobs. When I drew pictures of myself as an adult, I would draw a big cleavage line. Alone in my room at night, I would stuff some stress balls down my nightgown and coo, "Hello, boyyyyyyyyyyys."

Now that the universe* bestowed upon me the boobs of my dreams (*universe = Ashkenazi genes), they have become a big part of my identity. My breast development coincided with my popularity skyrocketing; whether they gave me more confidence or happened to appear when I became more confident is a mystery I never intend to solve. Having been boy crazy from a young age, I was delighted when the boys I pined for finally started to notice me, with my boobs drawing their eyes to my more important but subtler features, such as my smile and personality.

As I got older and gained weight/went on birth control, my boobs grew from a modest B to a "Why do I look skanky even in a T-shirt?" DD. Sometimes, they're big in a cartoonish way that doesn't feel like they're a part of my body. So, when I became a comedian, I had a choice: be objectified against my will *or* take charge of my image and show them off with an ironic brazenness. Think Jessica Rabbit sitting on the toilet during a shit attack. It's a mix of pride and apology, as if to say, "I know I look like this, but DON'T JERK OFF TO ME."

So, despite my own hmm/ugh/what?/yeah baby!/eh relationship with my breasts, I rarely think about the fact that, as Caitlin says, they could kill me. I got tested for the BRCA gene in the post-Jolie wave and was relieved to find that I was in the clear. But I realize how lucky I am, as this is not the case for an overwhelming number of women, especially those of Ashkenazi Jewish descent.

Every woman's experience with her boobs is specific and personal. As you read Caitlin's book, I hope that you reevaluate and appreciate your relationship with not just your boobs, but your body as a whole.

—Rachel and her boobs

INTRODUCTION

I had amazing twenty-eight-year-old breasts. They were huge, soft, and beautiful—I measured 32G, a fan favorite. But I hated them. I tested positive for the BRCA1 genetic mutation, specifically the 538insC BRCA1, which my doctors said gave me an 82 percent chance of getting breast cancer in my lifetime.[1] That statistic made me go 100 percent insane. It didn't help that I was born exactly nine months after my aunt Iris died of breast cancer at thirty-three years old. I was lovingly and terrifyingly welcomed into the world as her reincarnation. Growing up in my family, breast cancer was always the huge pink ribbon in the room.

I conquered these fears with the decision to have a preventative double mastectomy and share it with as many women as possible. I'm a comedian and a performer, and I can't be trusted with secrets, especially my own.

Sadly, I couldn't live-tweet the surgery. Fortunately, *Glamour* produced a docuseries that followed me through the very beginning of the process: *Screw You Cancer*. To date, it has more than 7 million views, was the first digital series to win a Television Academy Honor (Emmy Award), and won the National Magazine Award for Best Video. All I cared about at the time was trying to make my plastic surgeon laugh. There I was at twenty-eight, honestly sharing my experience with breast cancer prevention, BRCA, and a preventative mastectomy: a new spokeswoman with newer boobs. Most women who have mastectomies have had cancer or are typically older. I had a *double* mastectomy at twenty-eight without a cancer diagnosis. I call it the Angelina Jolie Surgery. It's like we are twins, or sisters, or best friends, but one of us is avoiding Brad Pitt and the other is avoiding her credit-card debt. After Jolie's *New York Times* op-ed piece in 2013, one study showed the number of women referred to genetic counseling increased by 85 percent. Additionally, the number of BRCA1/2 carriers identified increased by 107 percent after she went public.[2] Angelina opened the door to this world, but I am able to give you the grand tour. Until now, readers have been left to decode research journals or Google until three in the morning. I needed a place that wasn't just scientific and depressing. Oh hai! That's me! And this book will do just that.

Screw You Cancer covered the first half of my journey, and *Dangerous Boobies* is here to provide all the gritty details. Join me as I go from getting tested for BRCA to looking in the mirror at my mastectomy scars. You will travel with me as I confess and cry through my feelings to every woman in a Sephora. How do you talk to your family members about this? What about your significant other? How do you pick new nipples? How do your notions of femininity evolve or remain unchanged? How do you have sex after lying in bed for two weeks?

My story covers all of that—the funny, the gross, and the difficult in-betweens—from a girl who has already made you a friendship bracelet.

But enough about me (for now). Let's talk about you! Because we're in this together!

If you are at risk for the BRCA gene and are thinking of getting tested: Take your time and think some more. Assuming you don't have cancer, there is nothing to treat immediately. See a genetic counselor and find out the facts. Take it easy and be patient with yourself, and do only what you're ready for. It's your life, your decision—so lose the judgment that you're carrying around, and do what's best for you.

If you are positive for the BRCA gene mutation and are thinking of getting the surgery: First of all, don't be afraid. It will all be okay. I know if someone had said that to me, I wouldn't have believed them, and I would have thrown this book down and eaten my feelings. (Do order the French fries. They are delicious.) I understand completely if you are not ready for all of this yet. You can always pick it back up later when you are ready. Even reading this far was more than I could do when I was first diagnosed, so great job!

If you are reading this book to help a friend: Wow! You are so nice! What a good person you are! Thank you. Know that your support will help in more ways than you can imagine. Your being there is a big deal, and it is the reason we get dressed and out of bed, laugh again, and feel like a normal person during the process. And thank you in advance for the gossip magazines and ice cream, which are essential.

If you have had cancer or have it now and would like to read about my experience: I admire you so much. What I did will never be as difficult, and I am a wimp compared to you. I am terrified of cancer. I hope there is something in this book that you connect with and find comfort and humor in. Or you can use this book as a coaster for your morning green smoothie.

If you just want to see pictures of boobies: Whoa! I can't believe you read this far! That should be your quota for the week, right?! Is your Wi-Fi down? Did you already read every copy of *Playboy* cover to cover? I'm impressed you grabbed your older sister's copy of my book to quench your thirst! Go to page 232, you overachiever, you.

Whatever your reason for picking up *Dangerous Boobies*, you are not alone. That is the most important thing. Even if you want to be alone, which is understandable, you aren't far from someone who has gone through the same experience and has had the same difficult conversations with her family and friends. Yes, it is terrifying, but it doesn't have to be lonely. I did it alone for a while and had nothing to show for it but an unhealthy WebMD addiction. (I still have that, but let's deal with one issue at a time.)

If you are looking for this book to give you permission to have a double mastectomy—you have it! You have permission to do whatever the hell you want—it is your body. This is my experience, but you get to choose for yourself what you want for your beautiful body and your magnificent future.

I don't know exactly how to say "Let's hug" in book form. If we were next to each other right now, that tight, squeezing feeling that smells like Gucci 2 perfume would be me wrapping my arms around you. Instead, I'll just say, "Let's be friends." I'm not good at budgets, miniature golf, or handstands, but I am a great friend. And it's about to get personal. Like way, *way* personal. The kind of personal that's reserved for *gooooood* friends. As your friend, not only will I tell you everything you could ever want to know about the breast cancer gene and choosing new boobs, but I will also hold your hair back when you are sick, hate your exes without meeting them, and never speak of that one night in Greece. It will be great. Also, you should wear more blue. You look really good in blue.

Love,
Caitlin

HOOKER WITH A HEART

The photographer shook her head. "Yeah, there's lots of boob in that one too."

My entire life was filled with *lots of boob*. I angled my arms. I pulled my ribs back and my hips forward, as if Tyra were screaming at me from the sidelines of *America's Next Top Model*. I attempted to stick out my elbow and elongate my neck. I looked like a Cirque du Soleil du Reject, nothing worked.

The reality was that my boobs were taking over my life. This wasn't new; these tits loved to upstage me. Teen boys would yell at me from the street, weird men would follow me for a few blocks, and women would stare at me in shock. "How does someone so short have such huge boobs?!" I was always being asked the smartest questions.

To compensate, I wore scarves and layers to conceal my chest. It worked—I was (almost) able to stylishly drown my breasts and sexuality while simultaneously looking a little pregnant or homeless, or both.

Did my boobs hurt my back? Yep! Did they ruin every outfit I ever tried on? You betcha! Did they make me oversexualized at every event? Duh! These big little shits have been outshining me since eighth grade. From Chanukah parties to N'Sync concerts, the terrible twins just wouldn't quit.

And now they were taking over my photo session. I was supposed to be getting head shots taken for my acting portfolio, something that usually made me feel great. Hair and makeup and attention and more attention—sign me up! But this wasn't one of those '80s-montage makeover moments. We were in crisis mode. How do we hide these boobies? After three shirt changes and two bra changes, the photographer suggested, "Let's try a blazer?"

Just to clarify: A blazer is the kiss of death; wrap it up— game over. Nothing we tried could take attention away from my big boobies, so we were forced to cover and bury. My breasts successfully hijacked this photo session. All I needed was a microphone and a brick wall, and I was a middle-aged woman doing standup in the '90s. (To be fair, that is kinda a dream role.)

But the acting roles I was looking to be cast in didn't include my canyon of cleavage. I wanted to book a commercial for things like the Infinity Combo: Mop & Blender, and instead I looked like I would be cast as "Hooker #2 (with a Heart)" or "Ex-Wife Who's RLY into Margaritas."

Let's get real honest, real fast: I had size 32G boobs. I know—so big! G—as in GEE-THOSE-ARE-BIG G. Get-off-my-body G. Good-luck-hiding-those G. Why-would-God-punish-thee G! They were massive. Too big, Linebacker-Who-Likes-to-Bake Big. Boys loved them, girls wanted them, and friends couldn't believe I hid them so well. "Caitlin, there is NO way they are Gs!" I hated my boobs with all my heart. I made it my personal mission to keep them secured and camouflaged like the deadly weapons they were.

While we are being honest: They might one day have killed me. I tested positive for the BRCA genetic mutation, giving me a staggeringly high risk of developing breast cancer and ovarian cancer. #Blessed. This is a heredity-based mutation and in my case passed down from my father's Ashkenazi Jewish genes. I grew up in a Jewish-Catholic home, split fifty-fifty, and my top half was fully kosher. My father is the only living relative in his immediate family, and growing up I watched my favorite people lose battles with cancer. As a child, cancer was the monster under my bed. I would worry cancer would come for my sister or little brother. As I grew, I quickly became an expert at blocking out all feelings toward cancer. I just stuffed it down like a good little Catholic.

Massive deadly breasts that must be concealed? Someone make this movie. I would be happy to be cast in any production of anything actually, but I wanted to make the choice of what parts I could be in and not have my boobs make that decision for me. #RESIST. I also found myself apologizing the entire time during the photo shoot. I had lower self-esteem than that sad girl at the library you avoid making eye contact with. I was sorry it was such a concern, I was sorry that I was so unhappy with how I looked, and I was sorry my breasts were my biggest problem. I didn't want my miserable experience to rub off on the photographer. I was used to this struggle, but the photographer shouldn't have it wreck her day, too.

And then I was angry. This ruined my entire experience. Yes, I have body issues—I am a female actress, aren't I? Pile on my boob issues, and we were at an all-time high. And yes, I knew I needed more therapy, but whatever I did, the boobs were taking over my body and claiming it as their throne. I had no control over them. I know it's grating to be reading this if you are a woman with smaller breasts who wished you had bigger ones. It's like my friend Colin, who won't shut up about his huge hands—we get it. But living this way wasn't half as much fun as Colin's adventures.

My husband used to hold up my boobs when we would shower together to give my back a break. Girls with big twins, try it—it's amazing. It you don't have a shower buddy, use a shelf or counter. Just place the big twins on for a second, take a deep breath, and let your back relax. It's just the BEST. (But if you literally have twins who are children, don't leave them on a shelf or counter alone.)

My breasts would dictate what I could wear, how much I had to cover up, how I held my body, and how people would treat me. "Eyes up here, buddy. We're at a funeral. It's embarrassing." I would wear a compression bra and a tank top to help with cleavage spillage. Then I would top it all off with a V-neck T-shirt to avoid a uniboob. I couldn't control how people responded to my breasts, but I was going to do whatever I could to keep them on lock. Oh and I would wear a skirt or pants, whatever was clean, but even that didn't matter.

In college I considered getting breast-reduction surgery, but it all felt too intense. I was more comfortable hating my body. I was used to fourteen-year-old boys yelling "Big titties!" as they ran away giggling.

But that afternoon I was fed up. I wanted more control over everything: the photo session, my body, and my boobs. It didn't feel at all like I was representing myself. It felt like we were working with a disguise. I didn't want to play the parts my breasts could cast me in. And a head shot typically doesn't show your whole body. The eight-by-ten-inch photo cuts you right under your chest, right at your waist. For me, that would be 50 percent cleavage guaranteed.

Now, head shots are just a colorful requirement e-mailed to directors digitally (for some reason, everyone has *very blue* eyes). I miss the days when diners were filled with glossy black-and-white head shots of movie stars, actors, and the owner's cousin.

I have wanted to be a professional actress since I was three years old and was cast in a local *Magnum PI* commercial. The lights, the makeup, the free snacks—all of it delighted me, and I decided it would be my life. Then, in fifth grade, I was given one line as a Munchkin in *The Wizard of Oz*, and I understood this was my calling.

So I earned a bachelor of fine arts in acting and moved to New York. I even had some early success! I made a tiny cameo as Drunk Girl in Pirate Costume in the critically acclaimed blockbuster *Step Up 3D*. It required no hip-hop dancing.

Now I needed head shots—and I wanted photos that would increase my chances of being cast as anyone besides "Russian Hamster Smuggler."

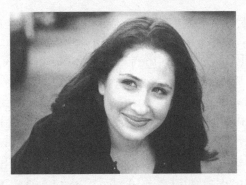

Pop quiz: How old am I in this photo? Thirty? Thirty-five? Nope. I'm *still* not thirty-five. That was me at twenty-one. Barely legal to drink, but I look like I'm going out for a district-attorney role in *Law and Order*. I had just dyed my hair black because I was in a loveless relationship and had the photographer crop the photo to hide the waterfall of cleavage.

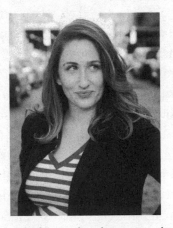

I'm twenty-eight here, looking a decade younger than my first head shot. Different hair; same blazer. I'm working my best face to compensate for my boobs. Signature look of not looking at the camera because I'm so uncomfortable, but like in a cute way.

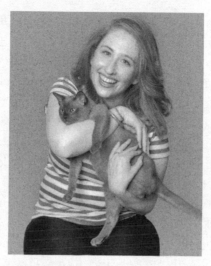

When in doubt, block your boobs with a cat! Show casting directors how good you are with miserable animals.

I had brought my favorite JLo album (*On the 6*) because I wanted to feel beautiful and weightless—"Feelin' So Good"! But my boobs brought me right back down to earth. I was distracted and demoralized, and I needed deodorant. The photo session ended: Boobs 2, Brodnick 0.

I rolled my suitcase away from the hip Meatpacking District studio over the romantically charming but heel-tripping cobblestone streets, feeling defeated. My hopes had been drowned by a blazer. I started to doubt my whole acting career. "Maybe this *is* all I can offer? Maybe I will just have to be cast as the Sexy Dog Walker or Pregnant Aesthetician?" I treated myself to a cab, sat back on the smelly pleather seats, and tried not to cry.

I wanted to escape my body. I wanted to propel my life into the future. I felt this way in middle school and college:

The next step was always going to be better. *Then* I will feel happier. *Then* I will be confident.

As I was crossing the Fifty-Ninth Street Bridge, I thought, "I cannot wait until I am sixty and I can get a mastectomy so I'm finally free of these horrible things." That was my first sobering thought.

My second one was, "Isn't life supposed to be amazing at twenty-eight? Aren't I in my prime? Or at least a *type* of prime?" And then I had an epiphany, or we hit a pothole, or I threw up in my mouth. I wanted to get the surgery—and I wanted to get it *now*.

It felt completely wild to give myself permission to jump into this extreme decision. I knew it was emotional—but let's be honest, every decision I make is emotional, and that isn't going to change anytime soon. It felt right, and for once I wasn't *as* scared.

Not only were my breasts subjecting me to blazers and hooker roles, but also . . . they might actually END me.

SUPERSERIOUS SIX-YEAR-OLD

My childhood was like every other kid's life in my Maryland neighborhood—I loved *Inspector Gadget*, swimming at the YMCA, and recess. Totally normal. Except for one little thing: Everyone. Kept. Dying.

One by one, my family members died of cancer. An aunt, another aunt, a grandparent or two or three . . . So, we talked a lot about death growing up. Didn't you? No? I was obsessed with death. When I would blow out my birthday candles and make a wish, I would wish for Andy to like me and for us be locked in a mall overnight and that my little sister wouldn't die. (I made my wishes in that order. I just *really* wanted to get locked in a mall with Andy.)

I didn't think this was unusual. I mean, Jewish people talk about death a lot. *A lot.* All of our holidays are focused on remembering the people who have died and how to avoid future deaths. No reincarnation or resurrection stories for us, just some good, simple death, to be celebrated every chance we get.

And on the days between holidays, we talk about the Holocaust. I knew every detail about how my uncle Charley's parents survived the Holocaust. When I was six years old, I explained to my cousin how "Charley's childhood was responsible for his detachment from the rest of our family." I filled her in while we were playing on our new swing set.

I was fascinated with death as a child, not cool Wednesday Addams or *The Craft* death obsessed, but like scared shitless, so I watched really cool shows like *Barney and Friends* and *Sesame Street* with my brother, who was ten years younger, because no one else ever died. (Except *Mr. Hooper.* But I blocked it out! I can't handle that type of instability!) I was always sitting with my aging grandparents wondering, "Is this the end?"

My father had two older sisters, Iris and Valia. In 1982 they were both living in California, looking for rich husbands, when Iris found a lump in her breast. Her mother, my Bubby, had just five years before battled breast cancer and had a radical mastectomy,* removing one of her breasts. Iris was twenty-eight years old and afraid, so she ignored it. You know what happened next. It grew as she kept going about her life. She had a lot going on. It was the '80s, and she had a solid group of friends, including Mike the Psychic, who, in retrospect, either wasn't very good or DEFINITELY should have spoken up. Iris had a life to live, and this bump in her breast wasn't going to stop her. It had grown to a dark round mass the size of a golf ball by the time she finally went to the doctor.

---

* According to Cancer.gov, a radical mastectomy is "surgery for breast cancer in which the breast, chest muscles, and all of the lymph nodes under the arm are removed. For many years, this was the breast cancer operation used most often, but it is used rarely now. Doctors consider radical mastectomy only when the tumor has spread to the chest muscles."

By then, like all tragic stories, it was too late. She immediately began aggressive treatment, with support from doctors and family, and tried her best to fight. As Iris received chemotherapy, everyone hoped for a successful recovery. Instead, she died abruptly from a blood clot due to treatment. She died in her mother's arms. She was just thirty-three.

The little Jewish family from Baltimore was wrecked. Sadness, pain, and anger were jumbled together in a grief cocktail they didn't know if they could survive. There were so many unfinished plans. My parents had been married for only a year. My grandparents had so many more meals to prepare for a full table. There were jokes that were never told and memories they were counting on having. She left everyone a little more alone.

And then—I was born! I came into the world oblivious: Oh, hhiiiiiiii!!! Were you guys crying? Sorry, I didn't notice. I pooped in my diaper while eating brownie batter—you have to figure out which is which!

As a small child, I understood that my family was sometimes sad, and I knew who Iris was, but I didn't have much patience for heavy hearts. I wanted to act out my favorite songs in *Grease*! I needed to practice aboveground synchronized swimming! I had imaginary farms to build, and puppets to talk to, and dresses to design out of napkins, and dirt to taste! I had to wear all of my Bubby's jewelry at the same time and eat SpaghettiOs before my dinner! *I know you are very upset and we might be lighting a candle to honor the dead, but right now I need someone to watch my jazz performance to Patti LaBelle's greatest hits! We are all very busy.*

There were dance recitals and Rosh Hashanah dinners where relatives would say, "Iris would have loved this matzo ball soup" or "Iris got Poppy so angry because she wouldn't stop giggling during the prayers." My sister and I did our best to giggle and create adequate disturbance to carry on her legacy. It was a very important job, and we were too hyped up on gefilte fish not to.

We were told the same stories over and over again. We knew them by heart. "Iris was everyone's favorite teacher at her school, she was writing a book, and she saved Valia's life when she was in a deep depression." No one ever fully recovered. Bubby kept everything of Iris's from ballet shoes to lip liner. She would have moaned, "Mom this is all wasted space," like we all say to our mothers who wish we grew up a little slower.

I was always told that I looked the most like Iris, which creeped me out. Guys—she was dead. I didn't want to look like a memory. There were many pictures of her, some when she was sick in a hospital bed, some when she looked very chubby and uncomfortable. I wanted to look like Kelly Kapowski from *Saved by the Bell*, but everyone made sure to tell me how much I looked like Iris, the *shaineh maidel*. They needed to. It made them feel like she was still there with them. But I needed to be reassured I would date Zach Morris and ride in a pink convertible in high school.

Meanwhile, my grandparents were children of immigrants fleeing Russia and survived the Great Depression, but neither could survive cancer. Of course, Poppy smoked for forty-two years. As soon as I was born, he quit cold turkey—his love beat nicotine! I can't even quit eating cold turkey, cold turkey. He managed to stop smoking overnight—but forty-two years is a long time, and even if he didn't suffer from lung cancer, he didn't escape it. Poppy died of pancreatic cancer when I was in tenth grade. His funeral was jam-packed. There was a line out the door of the funeral home, and traffic came to a halt. His funeral stopped Baltimore and the Brodnicks.

Luckily, I still had my Bubby. Bubby made me feel like I could do anything. I felt strong and daring, and safe. To have the world shut away when my Bubby and I were together was the greatest gift and the closest thing I came to meditation as a child. It was perfect.

Nothing I describe will come close to a tight, loving squeeze followed by a big, wet kiss planted directly into my ear and her laugh. My Bubby and I were a perfect pair, and she was proud to let everyone know it. "The Bubby and the Baby" they called us. Sure, she drove my mom crazy being perfectly passive aggressive at the same time as being overbearing, but Bubby's love was constant and smothering, the good type of smothering that makes you feel important.

After my Bubby's mastectomy she wore a prosthetic breast that fitted in a custom bra. I loved to squeeze her fake boob, and sometimes when it was laying around and she wasn't looking, I would punch it as hard as I could. Because kids love punching things.

And then, of course, her cancer came back when she was eighty-four, and it took her away forever. She died during my first year at college, but she waited until I came home for spring break and I could sing her to sleep one last time. Her death sent me into a deep sadness and a new sense of emptiness.

A light through all the heaviness was visits with my aunt Valia. We would sit at a coffee shop attached to the Barnes & Noble off Reisterstown Road. She would order me hot chocolate and a corn muffin, and we would discuss life like grown-ups. I would tell her what was happening in sixth grade: About how Jessa's mom didn't like that Kelsie and I were friends, because Jessa was Kelsie's friend first, but I thought Jessa's mom was maybe a closeted lesbian and so had other things on her mind. About the fact that Anna C. said I wasn't behaving like a true best friend and returned my friendship necklace I got her at Disney World and how it hurt but she was right.

And I would explain that I needed to move to New York City as soon as I graduated high school because I hated life in my town. For example: my crush Sebastian who ignored me and turned out to be a creep and had sex with two sisters, and both sisters said he had a small penis! And even though I had never actually seen a real penis, I knew it wasn't something I wanted to work with.

Valia loved all of it. She took my anxiety seriously, and she would encourage me to ignore the trashy bullies and introduced me to Audrey Hepburn, in hopes I would slow my roll. Instead, I became the weird theater girl who was always gazing far off into the corner of the gym, hoping someone would Sabrina her.

Valia was my father's older sister. She had lived in Baltimore her whole life and hated it too. She wanted to be a world-famous actress with all of the accompanying opportunities she never had in Baltimore. When she was first diagnosed with pancreatic cancer, she was given a six-month life expectancy and lived for another five years. After each round of chemo, she would be tired and distant. My sister, McKenzie, doubled down on her phone calls. We tried to eke out as many conversations as possible. Valia died of pancreatic cancer in 2009.

With each death, I felt a growing disconnect with my peers. I couldn't understand why they would argue or obsess over boys who looked nothing like Heath Ledger. (Later, I obsessed about the death of Heath Ledger.) Didn't they know that life was short and that none of this stuff mattered once we all inevitably got cancer? Didn't they know the end of life was imminent?

My friends seemed happy in their oblivion, but I couldn't shake the feeling that the ghost of doom was following me around, hiding in my locker, and waiting to pounce.

CANCER IS AN EMOTIONLESS BITCH WHO WILL RUIN YOUR BRUNCH PLANS

I am not a real doctor, and I am not even a fake doctor. But I am a big fan of doctors who understand the ever-changing data on heredity cancers. When I read a medical abstract, my anxiety flourishes. I see numbers and text that all look very serious and important, and then my dyslexia tells me "BECCA has a 45 degree risk of rental couch cancer." So I refer to my doctors and to genetic counselors and websites like the National Institutes of Health for the information I need to know.

What I do understand is that cancers are irregular cells that want to harm your body. In other words, cancer is a bitch who doesn't care if you are a nice person who just had lunch with your grandmother or helped a blind dog find its bone. There are many types of cancers, and all have their own teams of cells behaving badly. Like villains, they have gone rogue and refuse to follow the law of the land. All cells should follow a health code of when to live, when to grow, and when to die. Instead, cancer cells continue to grow and divide of their own free will. A normal cell stays put, whereas cancer cells might try to grow and develop in other parts of the body where they aren't welcome. These little tiny cells have a strong Napoleon complex, like that guy Phil from Advanced Placement French.* A normal body is pretty great at working to destroy unhealthy cells and naturally and automatically disposes of them. It is programmed to defend against villainous rogue cells with genes like BRCA. But if you have a mutation or a faulty gene, like I was born with, your body's forces are weaker against certain cancers. According to supersmart doctor Anne Marie McCarthy from Massachusetts General Hospital, "The uncontrolled cell growth in cancer cells is caused by mutations in the cell's DNA. Our body has several methods to fix mutations—including the proteins made by BRCA1/2 genes. When you have a BRCA mutation, the mutation fixing proteins do not work, so your body has one less tool to fix mutations that cause uncontrolled cell growth, and therefore you are more prone to getting cancer."

Being BRCA mutation-positive means you have a mutated version of one of the two BRCA (Breast Cancer) genes (I know, BRCA is a boring name, but at least it's not in Latin). We are all born with *BRCA1* and *BRCA2*, two different genes on different chromosomes that help suppress cancer from developing. If you have a mutation in one of the genes, your body is less able to fix mistakes in DNA, and an accumulation of these mistakes can lead to

---

* JK. I was in Beginner French for three years.

cancer. BRCA mutations make you more likely to develop breast, ovarian, and other cancers, and the risks are generally slightly higher with BRCA1 than with BRCA2. Both men and women can be positive for the BRCA gene and can pass it down to their children. A BRCA1/2 gene is not a virus or sickness you get over time. It is something you have as soon as you are born, like a full head of hair, blue eyes, or giggles during almost all serious events (like this girl!). Ashkenazi Jewish families have the highest rate of BRCA mutations, affecting one out of forty people.[1] In non-Jewish women, mutations are more rare (two to three per one thousand), which is why everyone does not currently get BRCA testing.

And it's not just the boobs that are targeted. Melanoma, pancreatic, and prostate cancer risks are all increased in families who are BRCA positive.[2] My Poppy and Valia died from pancreatic cancer, and my Bubby and my aunt Iris both had breast cancer. My father has regular screenings for prostate cancer and all of the above because he's ON TOP OF HIS SHIT.

I'm not an oncologist. But I am a storyteller, which is definitely why I prefer to think of cancer as a villain, a DC Comic villain, to be specific. All cancers/villains have one goal: to destroy Superman. (In this world, I am Superman, because it's my story and I make the rules.) Superman has to always be aware of the bad guys lurking in dark alleys or in business suits and has to find the best tools to fight the criminals trying to take him down.

Bad guy Doomsday will always attack Superman with brute force, for example. Like most cancers, Doomsday needs to be destroyed with an equal or stronger power, like chemotherapy and radiation. All hands on deck to destroy this cancerous evildoer.

Lex Luthor is a hereditary cancer and more of an insidious villain. This guy is intelligent and conniving, dressed in a sharp suit. To beat him, Superman has to outsmart him, playing a complex game of genetic chess better than Luthor does in order to survive.

While we're at it, Silver Banshee is ovarian cancer, because she blends and hides and then strikes suddenly.

Kryptonite is cigarette smoke, because sometimes you want a little puff when you are on vacation, but that shit stick will ultimately destroy you.

Pancreatic cancer is Gorilla Grodd—because of course it is.

These metaphors work for me, though I hate cancer so much that I feel guilty giving it cute comic-book names. Because cancer doesn't deserve it. There are no snazzy costumes, no redeeming qualities, no sidekicks with bright colors and funny catchphrases. There is no commercial break, and the fighting doesn't stop after the submarine explodes in act 3.

Plus, I am actually not at all like Superman. I am not a hero, and I am not brave and bold in the face of deathly danger—I am afraid of cancer, and I don't want to battle anything stronger than a sleeve of Girl Scout cookies. But I don't have much of a choice, and when I have to put on a cape and tights and eyeliner, that's what I do.

THERE ARE NO DUMB QUESTIONS, JUST DUMB GIRLS WHO REFUSE TO GO TO THE DOCTOR TO ASK QUESTIONS

Because my dad is the only surviving member in his family, he was hungry for information. He was smart, and he went on the hunt for a genetic connection. There had to be a reason an entire family was wiped out by cancer. It had to be more than bad luck, right?

He started working with John Hopkins Hospital as a research patient. That's where he was told about the new discovery of a cancer-related genetic mutation. He was elated to learn about it—he had been right, there was something happening to his family, and he could finally make sense out of all this sickness and pain. It wasn't just a coincidence! And because there was a link to these cancers, maybe there would be a cure?

No surprise, my dad tested positive for BRCA1. My mom didn't bother getting tested—she is a hot blonde shiksa with a body that won't quit and no family history of breast or ovarian cancer. With zero family history of these cancers and a Welsh-Scottish-Catholic background, she isn't at risk for the gene. But my dad's gene was passed down from his very Jewish genes, and there was a chance his children would have it too. My brother and sister and I had a fifty-fifty chance of testing positive. My dad wanted us to get tested immediately. I refused.

I love my dad—and he's really smart and I appreciated his fears—but I was twenty-one and I was NOT GETTING ANY TESTING DONE, THANKS. Why would I want that information? I was already afraid of my own life ending. Why did I need evidence to take away any speck of hope that I might actually survive to a reasonably old age? Lemme keep that, okay? And don't the risks of cancer rise as you get older anyway? Great. Let's worry about it when I'm older. Much older.

Plus, my life was finally getting good, and I didn't want to muck with that. I fell asleep eating pizza in bed and woke to the sounds of New York City outside my minuscule apartment window. I was a free woman. And I just met this *really* cool guy! His name is Allen. He is a free thinker, a smart man who wants to change the world, and I want to be a part of that. We just graduated college and are going to take over NYC. We have too much to live for, and cancer is *not in the equation.*

Oh, and even if I were gung ho on getting the test— which I definitely was not—did I mention I suffer from Vasovagal Syndrome? Don't know what that is? I'll tell you. It sounds like delicious Austrian pastry meant to be eaten with jam, but no. Having a vasovagal response (neurocardiogenic syncope) means my body is triggered when I see my own blood and sometimes needles. It causes my blood pressure to drop until I get light-headed and dizzy, and my body starts to sweat and I throw up. Every time I need a shot, nurses rush over with ice packs for my neck and let me lay down with my feet above my head, and we wait it out. I am fun, guys—invite me to all your parties! This makes doctor appointments very uncomfortable for all involved, so I avoid all blood work if possible.

My sister took the blood test for BRCA one spring break when she was home from college, because of course she did. She is great at that stuff. She always writes something sweet and special in birthday cards, instead of my classic lines, like "U B so GR8." Once again, she was being the perfect daughter and getting a test that my parents cared so much about.

And guess what?! She was negative for the gene! NEG-ATIVE! As in, *does not have the gene mutation, does not have to worry, does not have a higher risk of breast cancer, and does not have to give it another thought.* My brother was far too young to have the test taken and could focus on important things like playing lead guitar in his high school punk band.

I still wasn't having it. My family pushed me for years, but I was obstinate. My dad had even bought me one of the first DNA testing kits—one that used a swab instead of a needle. The overpriced kit would let me swipe a cheek, mail it in, and wait for results, with little to no stress. But I wasn't handing over any swabs just yet. I kept that kit behind the closed doors of my overstuffed closet under a pile of Halloween wigs. *I hated that kit.* It just sat there, waiting, with its passive-aggressive whispers of impending doom.

Growing up, we had the identical family pattern as my father's: two older sisters and a younger brother. We were always told that we reminded everyone of my father's sisters, and we were just as close. My child-size logic explained that if we were just like his family, the second daughter—my sister, McKenzie—would die of cancer at thirty-three. This is morbid and intense for a child to deduce, but there I was, making comparisons and preparing for my doomed future. I would ask my parents about her: Would she get sick? Would she die? How can we be sure?

I did everything I could to keep her safe. I protected her on the school bus from bullies. I yelled in mean girls' faces when they called her names, and I would push any boy who wouldn't be her valentine. And as adults, I made sure her friends were treating her nicely and not expecting she walk their dogs for free. Her time was valuable.

McKenzie's negative results helped stoke my parents' fire—like if a gasoline can was used to stoke the fire. My family was amped! "See, Cait? You might be negative! You might not have it! You never know!"

I didn't want to know. I wanted to start a new chapter in my life. I wanted to try to get my comedy career off the ground, write a one-woman show. I had just joined a new improv team. I wanted to take job risks, not medical risks. In fact, I'd just decided to quit one of my many part-time jobs as a receptionist in a doctor's office so I could devote my energy to my own auditioning career full-time.

The doctor's office wasn't awful, but I couldn't take it anymore. It specialized in treating Broadway dancers, and I was in charge of booking their appointments, answering phones, and filing insurance claims. Performers would come in and leave, going back to their happy, fulfilling careers, while I was put on hold for hours at a time so I could argue over thirty-dollar reimbursements.

My favorite part of the job was when I could take a bathroom break. The handicap bathroom was a glorious oasis during a dark and smelly time. I would hide magazines in the medicine cabinet and spray down the stalls with Febreze and just have a little time alone. Then, after a little bit, but not long enough to cause concern, I would walk back to my desk, plaster on a smile, and try not to stab myself in the eyes with pens.

I said no to the test and yes to freedom. I was in charge! I was not going to be the one sashaying out the doors of life so soon. I had plans! I would be a freelance writer (not sure what I'd write about just yet) and audition on the side and live my life as a performer in New York City. The world was mine!

Except health insurance wasn't. Or it wouldn't be, if I quit my day job. And that's what finally made me take the test. The closer I came to leaving the gig and going full-blown starving actress, the more I worried about my health. Before I officially quit, I decided I'd get those buzz-killing genetic tests taken. Plus, remember that great guy I met, the coolest, smartest, nicest person in the world? We just got engaged! So maybe it was a good time to check if I had a high risk of dying? As you do. I made an appointment with my doctor.

When I finally decided to get the official genetic test to see if I was positive for the BRCA mutation, I did it in the worst way possible. I should have researched genetic counselors who specialize in testing and the impact that has on your psyche, emotions, and future. Instead, I did the quicky-mart, express-lane, bootleg version and made an appointment with my general practitioner, the one who treated me for bladder infections and gave me flu shots. I might as well have gone to a podiatrist for an eye infection.

In my defense, I kinda liked my doctor. She was always late and sweaty, and she wobbled when she walked. I started seeing her only because she was part of a hospital group downtown and was close to one of my many part-time jobs. She laughed at two of my jokes and took my need for anti-depressants seriously, so she'd do. Plus, she had an auntie vibe that made me feel like at any moment she would offer me a tray of cannoli.

I went to my doctor and first asked for a blood test to see if I had a gluten allergy, the most popular allergy in 2010. And then I said, hey, while she was in there getting some of my blood, could we just see if I have any genetic mutations that could alter the course of my life? Just for funzies? Before I could finish telling her my family history, she had ordered the blood test. I was of Ashkenazi descent, my aunt had breast cancer before she was fifty, and my father was positive, all red flags for increased likelihood for BRCA. So I was a great candidate. *Finally, I was cast in something.*

So I gave her my blood, and almost passed out like I always do, and rode the subway home alone, like I always do. I treated myself to a strawberry Pop-Tart, which wasn't gluten free. And then I felt relieved to tell my family I finally did it. I took the test, and now we can all Move On.

Well, not quite yet. That week, I was supercool and thought about the test results only about sixty-five times a day. It was impossible not to imagine how our lives would change if I tested positive. How would Allen react? Would my father feel guilty? Would this mean I would have to live the rest of my life in doctors' offices? That week I baked a lot of challah and talked about my feelings to any bodega cat that would listen.

Then I got a phone call and was told I needed to come into the office to go over my results with a surgeon from the hospital. It was routine, the woman on the phone assured me, and told me not to worry.

NOT TO WORRY? Too late, lady. I have been worrying for years! No plan on stopping! The new doctor I'd be meeting with handled all breast-related cases, and supposedly this was just precautionary. Still, I wasn't amped.

I was told to go to the east wing of the hospital, which was colder and more serious and there were no promises of cannoli. I went alone and checked in with the receptionist, who was so buried under file folders she could barely see my face, and waited in a room with old chairs, *Prevention* magazine, and cancer patients. I tried my hardest to focus on my postvisit Pop-Tarts.

I don't want to seem dramatic or too emotional, but for efficacy let's just call the breast surgeon *This Bitch* for the remainder of the story, shall we? So *This Bitch* came into the exam room like she was opening the New York Stock Exchange trading floor. Guns blazing and ready to wreak havoc on some fresh test results. She had a short haircut that belonged in the '80s, with shoes to match.

This Bitch proceeded to tell me everything she would recommend we do if I was positive for the BRCA mutation. "First thing, we would cut off your breasts." First thing? That's the very first thing? Why not ask me any questions?

Am I pregnant? Do I want to have this surgery? Have I sniffed glue? Do I think Justin Bieber and Selena Gomez are ever getting back together? Literally anything?

All *This Bitch* focused on was reciting her extensive mastectomy résumé. How great she was at surgery and how she performed them "all the time." She had another office in Pennsylvania or in Connecticut, where she preferred to operate, but that was to be worked out later, I think. I can't remember, because I had emotionally blacked out at this point.

This Bitch then left the room to go get the test results. I had a second to text my mom that I was in the doctor's office and waiting to hear the test results and made sure to add, "this doctr sux." I sat there alone, sweating through my skirt, trying not to cry.

This Bitch swiftly reentered, ready to rip off any Band-Aid in sight. Then she told me I was in fact BRCA1 positive. She added that I have a very high risk of breast cancer and handed me a few worksheets. Then she said she would leave me alone for a few minutes. And then *This Bitch* walked the F out of the room. SHE LET ME SIT THERE ALONE AND TERRIFIED. Like I was just dropped off at a sleep-away camp that moonlights as a horror-film set.

I called my mom and immediately started sobbing. It felt like I was telling her I was going to die. All of our family's fears were coming true. I cried and had flashbacks of everyone I lost to cancer. Valia had just died of pancreatic cancer. We had just buried her the year before, and now I had more hard evidence that cancer was coming for me next. My father's nightmare had come true: He had passed down the BRCA mutation and now had to worry he could lose his daughter.

It felt like the room was getting smaller and my future was doing the same. Then *This Bitch* walked in and asked me, "How are we doing?" We? Excuse me! Not so great, you sad, tired version of Sally Jessy Raphael! *We* are dealing with some deep shit here. *We* are not having a hard time picking out Froyo toppings. *We* are living a nightmare, and *we* have our mother on the phone who is at home weeping into her mixed-green salad.

This Bitch tried to say other things to me, but I was in an emotional blurry tunnel. Procedures were mentioned, and then I was given a folder and told to book a follow-up appointment for surgery with the receptionist outside. *This Bitch* left, to go perform all her mastectomies she was so fond of.

I could barely leave the exam room, but once I did, I just kept walking. Past the receptionist, who was still hiding under mounds of papers, down the elevator, through the exit, onto the street, where I called my mom back for the next cry.

I asked my mom to tell my dad because I couldn't bear it. I knew it was one of the hardest things I could have asked her to do, but I couldn't say the words to him. It was as if we were finally caught, as if cancer had followed us all, hunting and haunting us all our lives, and now it was sitting closer than ever.

Cancer wasn't just circling the block this time. It was on my doorstep, telling me I had only a few years before it was coming for me. It was an absolute horror, something I wasn't ready for at all. Our biggest fears were here on my chest. I was in a fog. I thought of my future, my family, my funeral.

But wait! This wasn't a cancer diagnosis; it was just a genetic mutation. Why did it feel like I was diagnosed with cancer? Cancer had stolen my loved ones and deprived me of Passover parties, sleepovers, and belly laughs. It was right there, tapping on my window. I had to keep repeating to myself, *I don't have cancer, I don't have cancer.* But it barely helped. I was consumed.

That night I went home and cried more to my family members on the phone and more to Allen. I did some light Googling on breast cancer prevention. And then I went to bed.

I didn't know what else to do, really. All I knew was that there was no way in hell I was going back to that hospital. I was getting as far away from *This Bitch* as I could, and I was never, ever going to get a double mastectomy.

I AM PATIENT-ZERO PATIENCE

I really, really hate mammograms. I know they are important and have saved many women's lives, but they suck. I hate that the well-meaning nurse tries to flatten your breast like a pancake as if you don't have any nerves running through it. It makes me pity Play-Doh. After the flattening free-for-all, I feel angry. I don't want my boobs to be analyzed and poked at and squished. I don't even want to wait around for the results. I just want to be in bed watching Japanese reality shows on Netflix.

I had my first mammogram immediately after my BRCA diagnosis. I booked the appointment and prayed they wouldn't find anything. The nurse took multiple pictures and then stopped and adjusted my breast, by pressing it down harder than I thought was humanly possible. Took some more shots, made adjustments, and continued. Every moment was chartable on a spectrum from uncomfortable to brutally painful. I should never have complained about my head shots.

Then I was told to stay and wait while they review "something on the X-ray." WHAT? I can't just *leave*? There was something to *review*? Is this an okay time to start crying? Because I am.

I was told my breasts were dense and this is common for most young women and that my young, dense breasts had bumps similar to breast cancer lumps. So, to have a better look, they would need to schedule an MRI to get a closer look. And now I hate MRIs.

Of course, I completely freaked out that they were lying to me and that I already had cancer. How big would this cancer be? Would it be in an advanced stage, since this was my first-ever mammogram? What would I tell my friends and family? Would I beat it, or would I die young, like my aunt had? What flowers will they have at my funeral, and will my cousin's ex-boyfriend come to my funeral? Is it too early to send invites? My brain can spin quickly into this downward spiral.

I tried to be a good sport. I really did. I made the appointments. I even showed up for them. But before the MRI was taken, they had to insert a contrast dye in my veins, via IV drip, so the tissue would be more easily captured by the MRI. You know what that means.

As soon as I saw the needle, I started to feel dizzy and prepared myself to throw up. I dry-heaved into the nearby sink. Great start! The patient nurses gave me fifteen minutes for my body to relax and my (old faithful) vasovagal response to dwindle. I felt my entire body start to sweat, and I fully drenched the hospital gown.

Finally, I was ready for the MRI. I lay facedown in a white claustrophobic tube and was told to relax. It felt like I could be compressed at any moment into a full-body mammogram. There were built-in holes in the tube that my breasts hung through, dangling toward the floor. It was embarrassing enough to be on top during sex and have my breasts flopping around without a care in the world, but at least Allen was into it. Here they were hanging down like two udders waiting to be relieved. Picture a robotic cow.

I tried to remain as calm as possible while I ground my teeth and listened to a series of clicks and typical loud-machine noises. I just wanted it to be over. What if I had to pee and couldn't hold it and peed all over the machine, causing an electrical fire? Or worse—what if I sneezed, ruined the images, and they would have to start all over?

By the time I finished my third emergency fantasy, it was over. The technicians said the films were clear and readable, and I would hear the results in about a week. I think they said something kind, too, but my mind was blurry. I just wanted to be back in my bed and sleep the stress away.

I spent the next week waiting for a call, saying mistakes were made and I for sure had cancer. I replayed all my greatest hits of worst-case scenarios. Would they call in the middle of an improv rehearsal where I was pretending to give birth inside a volcano? I would think about how I would tell my parents and if they would be strong for me when I couldn't. I thought about how the news would destroy my father and how much he had already lost. I wondered if people would give me a pass to stay home and cry myself to sleep if I had cancer. I thought about how horrible this would be to Allen and how much stress it would put on our relationship.

Would it be a single-lump cancer like Iris's, or would it quickly spread like a spiderweb to my other organs? I knew enough to be terrified, and I did a good job of it. I was even worried about how much I was worrying.

In the end, I was told I had "no cancer"—my breasts were fine. But I wasn't.

GOOGLE'S LAND OF HORRORS

It was four in the morning, Allen was asleep, the house was quiet, and no one could see what I was doing. It was the perfect time to WebMD.

WebMD is my kinky porn fetish. I do it alone, I don't want anyone else to know about it, and it's a habit I refuse to break. I know there are others like me, but I've kept this dirty secret to myself until now. I research every sickness, every toe fungus, every disease I could catch while back-packing in Bali. I am an independent woman, and if I want to read about ear discharge for two hours, I will.

Google is the most fun way to quietly torture yourself from the safety of your own home. With WebMD you are always one click away from a heart-pounding realization you have been living with a life-threatening disease since kindergarten. Actually, you might already be dead and not even know it. It's my emotional Russian roulette. One click and you can discover that your organic corn is a mutant crop that might kill you from the inside. Before I compare and contrast vaginal rejuvenation surgeries, let me read this quick article on the kneecap liposuction. Usually, I just hunt around, but this time my fetish had a purpose. I wanted to do as much research as possible on breast cancer prevention. Here we go—I finally have an excuse to search WebMD for helpful and relevant advice!

I couldn't do it. I tried, night after night, but I would usually lose focus and start rewatching *30 Rock* episodes. My attention for BRCA research dwindled to a flaky, ferocious four minutes, my worry would rise, and then I would pine to be distracted by the newest celebrity-endorsed pumice stone.

I finally broke up with WebMD—I wasn't even sure we could still be friends.

A few months and a few panic attacks later, I confessed to my dad casually over the phone that I had been avoiding my cancer screenings since my MRI episode.

"Oh, Cait, that's really not safe," he said quietly. His voice was different this time. It wasn't nagging or pushy; he was actually scared. I didn't want to go but I really didn't like the fear in his voice, so I made an appointment with a human. I collected my courage and went to see a genetic counselor. I met with one BRCA research scientist and one genetic counselor, and I was proud to show them my paperwork and the highlighting I had done to my WebMD printouts (mementos from the prebreakup days).

I was sure I would be given a gold star for my impressive research and was hungry for any type of validation. I quickly explained I understood I needed to avoid carcinogens, cut out animal products, and have babies before thirty to lower my risk of breast cancer. I had been vegan now for a total of four difficult days, and I was ready to prevent cancer.

"Wow, I can really see you did your homework," said the counselor, like a proud grandfather. I felt warm and fuzzy and smart. "But the lifestyle changes you've made aren't necessarily associated with genetic-based cancer. Being a vegan is very healthy, but it won't change your risk for this type of cancer."

Excuuuuse me?

They explained that in my case, my chances of developing breast cancer were based on my DNA. My BRCA mutation is something I was born with. So my chances of developing cancer are more likely based on the inherited BRCA mutation and not necessarily just from environmental and nutritional factors.

Are you *kidding me?* I was researching *the wrong kind of breast cancer?* Who even knew there was more than one cause of breast cancer? Also, WHERE'S MY BURGER?! SOMEONE GET ME A HOT DOG WRAPPED IN BACON!

Clearly, I had no idea what I was talking about. It didn't matter how many pages I highlighted. I needed to listen to this man—he knew how to help me.

We went over my risk factors. We went over how my risk of breast cancer would slowly increase over time and how my ovaries were also at high risk.[1] I would have to receive biyearly screenings, and my body would be monitored. I would also be tested annually to see if I had any irregular results that could be a marker for ovarian cancer.

Because I was at high risk for cancer, I was able to have screenings typically not available to someone my age or someone cancer free. It was almost as if my medical folder was red-flagged and I was able to go to the head of the class. I would be given access to in-depth screenings, and doctors would treat my medical conditions with the awareness of my new diagnosis.

I listened as hard as I could, trying to memorize everything the genetic counselor said. I had to later explain all of this to Allen and parents and to anyone I passed on the street, and I didn't want to mess it up. I started to sweat through my wrinkled collared shirt. Never. Not. Sweating.

I was told that some women choose surgical procedures, like a preventative mastectomy or removing the ovaries (oophorectomy). The incredible medical oncologist, and clinical investigator, Dr. Payal Shah explained to me, "We recommend oophorectomy after completion of child-bearing, but by age forty in BRCA1 carriers and by forty to forty-five in BRCA2 carriers. Breast-feeding doesn't really come into play unless women *want* to keep their breasts in so that they can breast-feed." If I chose to have a prophylactic (preventative) double mastectomy, doctors would remove all of the tissue and glands inside the breast, leaving just the pectoral muscle and skin. That procedure would significantly lower my chances of breast cancer. I could also choose nonsurgical options, like aggressive screenings and medications like Tamoxifen.[2] I was okay with the screenings, but I didn't like the idea of taking these pills for the next five years. Plus, if a medication doesn't have a corresponding commercial that includes an aging couple soaking in individual bathtubs, I'm not interested.

Still, I was relieved to hear I wouldn't need to be cut open right away and that I had more choices besides surgery. If I faint at the sight of needles, I could only imagine my reaction to a surgical scalpel. It was way more information than I was expecting, but somehow I felt more comfortable after that visit than I had since I'd gotten my test results.

I asked my genetic counselors my favorite question: What would you advise your sister or mother to do if she was diagnosed? Let's make this personal, because I am not some statistic. What would you tell someone you loved more than anything else in the world?

"Prophylactic mastectomy reduces the risk of breast cancer by more than 90 percent. Prophylactic oophorectomy has a similar effect on the risk of ovarian cancer and also reduces the risk of breast cancer."[3] Oophorectomy not only has a risk reduction for ovarian and breast cancers, but is also associated with lower risks of dying from breast cancer and ovarian cancer.[4]

I was proud of this question. But my doctors were taken aback and slightly uncomfortable. It was hard for them to answer, and instead they explained what they would do for their own bodies. They both said most doctors would probably opt for the surgery because they hate being patients. They don't like to have their time taken by appointments and waiting for results, and they would rather be in control. They didn't exactly answer my question, but that's okay.

That is not me. I was sure I could handle the nonsurgical, heavy-surveillance path. I am a great student. I like being around smart people in lab coats. I can totally do screenings twice a year. This girl does *not need surgery.*

I said thank you so much, took home my folder of information, and then canceled every single doctor's appointment he had recommended, like the great patient that I was.

I reported my visit back to Allen and my parents that I was under good care, and then I got drunk for three years.

THE GREAT FROSTY GLASS

I met Allen a month after we both graduated from college. We went to the same school, graduated the same year, in the same major, and had mutual friends, but he and I never spent any time together. I didn't know him, but I was friendly with his ex-girlfriend, whom I helped through their breakup because I was such a good friend and I am excellent at shitting on strangers to comfort my friends.

Then I met Allen and understood why his ex was so heartbroken. Of course his ex was crushed—he is the shit. He is the coolest person I have ever met. I would be devastated too. He is a gold mine of a person and great in bed. I mean, COME ON.

I met Allen and knew I wanted him in my life forever. I was willing to take whatever he was comfortable with, and luckily he liked me back. Allen is incredible. He is a sensitive feminist who volunteers twice a week, one day at a soup kitchen and one day at a home for previously incarcerated women. He grew up in a sad, scary household, around wild drug-addicted adults who were unsafe and emotionally abusive. He came out of that hell as one of the sweetest, most loving people I will ever meet. And I get to keep him.

I look up to him because I trust his judgment and because he's taller than I am. He helps me with grammar, taxes, and finding my keys. And he never judges me when I fart. I love all his different laughs: I love his shock-with-excitement laugh; his ironic-appreciation laugh; his giggle laugh; the laugh he shared with his grandmother; his silent, hysterical gasping-for-breath laugh; and the sweet one that turns into "aww" at the end.

We are very different—I make fast, strong decisions and worry about the cleanup later, while he is slow and methodical—but without him I would probably be selling meth on a riverboat. And so I married him.

Now I was newly married, happy, and terrified because I was BRCA1 positive. Breast cancer felt closer. I didn't want to be a cancer patient—I didn't want to be a patient at all.

With this diagnosis, I was told I should have screenings every six months. I didn't want to sit in the waiting room with people having chemotherapy and getting screenings. I didn't want to be a part of that club. I wanted to run away and become someone else. I ran into the loving arms of HGTV and Häagen-Dazs and stopped all medical appointments. And then I got drunk, real drunk. I always loved to drink with friends at parties, and I think every conversation I started that year was, "Oh and I have the BRCA gene, so my risks for dying of cancer are incredibly high and I might get cancer one day." I was more likely to have people slowly back away from me during a conversation than get cancer at that point. I was scared, emotional, and selfish. I took any opportunity I could to check out and escape my reality.

Being BRCA positive was the perfect excuse for me to get trashed. It was still a relatively new mutation and not many people understood it, so when I said my cancer chance was alarmingly high and I needed a drink, who was to stop me? I would say witty words with a big smile, and that was my ticket to drink for the rest of the night. Everyone wants to get a drink for a girl who might, maybe, could possibly, might, you never know, die of cancer.

It's recommended to have one glass of red wine a night for health, but I took it to a whole new expert alcoholic level. I wanted to sign out of life. I'll just sit this one out. You guys go ahead with your reality; I'm going to get comfortable with a bottle of white wine. White wine that I would freeze and suck out of the bottle like a CHAMP. I called the alcoholic Slurpee "slushy wine." It is still the best thing I have ever invented. I was fun, right? Right?! Isn't this what you do in college, or a few years after college, or when everyone else has real jobs, or just on a Tuesday night?

I used my diagnosis as the perfect excuse to party hard and get wasted. Who could stop me? I was a fun girl with a great sob story. I could drink my fears under the table because *"I deserphed thiiiiiiis."*

The first week after I was diagnosed, I went to my improv class, taught by the incredible Chris Gethard. Before class started, I told one of my friends about my results and began to cry, and every single girl in the class came over to offer me comfort and support. We all hugged and felt closer than ever, and then we did an improv scene about a donkey shopping for a bathing suit.

The diagnosis was still so new that I barely understood what I was talking about. I just knew that I should be worried. After class I went home and drank a few more cocktails of pinot grigio and 7Up.

Every comedian I know is afraid they will wake up one day and lose their "funny." That suddenly the world will figure out that they have been just screwing around this whole time, having a blast, and get caught one day empty-handed, without a joke to save their lives. Or that suddenly, they will be old and washed up, before they even have a chance to do a national Hanes underwear commercial.

Fear shut me out, it kept me home, and it isolated me from everyone I thought was talented and wanted to work with. Suddenly, I was convinced no one wanted to hang out with me and would bully myself to "just stay home; no one cares if you make it to the party—you're not that fun." With these loud fears, I wasn't able to make any simple decisions, and I wanted to hide. So I did. Facebook is great for that—you can post stupid photos and funny phrases, and everyone thinks you are fine. And I was very far from fine.

Cancer was all I could think about. When people would ask me how I was doing, I blurted back "I am BRCA POSITIVE!" and assailed them with the likelihood of my premature death. Oh, did you say something about you? I'm sorry—I can't focus on anything but myself.

Myself and the drinks menu. My life was hard, and it was going to get harder, so I might as well just enjoy myself and have six more beers. I was a fun drunk—until I wasn't anymore. My sad thoughts and I would curl up on my couch, have some dinner (gummy bears and wine), and watch TV until I passed out. I would try to stop drinking for two weeks, and once I even stopped for one hundred days, but as soon as I started up again, I became a garbage person who would repeat this pattern every two weeks.

I would find excuses to drink with my friends, reasons we all *needed* this girls' night out to get obliterated. Like because it was Friday, or getting cold outside, or the *Bachelor* season finale was disappointing. I was a master of excuses. I wanted everyone around me to be just as wasted, because "tonight is going to be the best night of our lives!"

I became anxious about where my second and third drinks would come from before I had a chance to finish my first. I could order two drinks at a time, with my third on deck. And you better believe I would resent the waitress if my glass wasn't filled to the top. Pour it UP! Pour it UP!

I drank to shut out the fear. I drank to shut out my voice in my head saying I wasn't good enough. I drank because I was jealous of someone's talent, body, Twitter followers. I drank because I had a bad day and because maybe you had a bad day. I wanted to make sure everyone in the room was drinking, I pushed drinks on everyone else to guarantee we all had a great night.

Pot? Sure, I will just do a little. I have a great impression of a dancing tuba. Lemme show you after this hit.

I was also an expert at morning-after apologies and making up for the havoc I caused while drunk. The only person I usually harmed was Allen. We would ride the subway home, and that's when the shit hit the fan, or I hit the fan—the side of the wall, the table, trash cans. I was out of my mind.

To most friends I was going through a hard time. It was "understandable," but it was also selfish, insane, and a waste of everyone's time and energy.

I sat at home and drank because:

I was mad I had the gene.
I was happy I didn't have cancer.

I was worried my kids would have to see their mother
   go through breast cancer.
I wasn't allowed to give my bartender a makeover.
I was scared I would ruin Allen's life.
I was afraid to get a mammogram.
I wasn't a Real Housewife. I hated myself.

When I did go out, my friends thought I was crazy fun.
Then I would get in a cab home and arrive at my apartment
just in time for all of the alcohol to hit me like a wave of
boozy bricks. Sometimes I would have to get out of a cab to
puke or choose to walk alone so I could pee on the side of the
street. I fell and hit my head, and then I did it again. There
was the time I couldn't remember where I lived and the
time I needed Allen to hold me up, *Weekend at Bernie's* style.

At every wedding I attended after college, I would binge
drink, puke in the bathroom, order another chardonnay,
and get back on the dance floor. I once was escorted out of
a male strip club during my best friend's bachelorette party
because I was too drunk to stand and the bouncer was sick
of holding me up. I thought he was just flirting with me.
I was not cute. I was selfish and very dangerous.

I would be stubborn and indignant to the people who
were closest to me. I would lash out like a bitchy monster
with a lot of feelings and reasons you should listen to her.

The first time I got drunk, I was mean to my little sister,
who was trying to help me when I was puking. The last
time I got drunk, I was mean to my husband for trying to
save my life.

One night when I drunkenly promised the bartender
I'd help him find his dream (my go-to drunk promise), he

gave me eight to twelve free sangrias, I smoked a cigarette, tried to steal a Christmas tree, paid double for said tree, hailed a cab, puked in the cab, and puked on the tree. The cab driver called the police because I was throwing my body around the cab and he thought I was throwing objects at him. I arrived at my apartment, waking Allen up in the middle of the night. He had to pay off the cab driver, to save me from being arrested. Then the cops and an ambulance rushed me to the hospital because I was unresponsive. I was a real peach.

This night was exactly two months after our wedding day, and if Allen wasn't home, I might have died. Instead, I woke up in the hospital after being treated for alcohol poisoning. Allen was in a chair next to my bed, his face white as a ghost. He had spent the whole night by my side, where it just so happened to be one of the busiest nights in the emergency room. People were coming and going with horrible bloody injuries, yelling that they were dying. He had to listen to the chaotic symphony of beeps and alarms as the emergencies poured in, while I slept through it in a drunken stupor, like a toxic baby in la-la land.

When I finally came to, Allen was white as a ghost, exhausted, and beaten down. I knew at that moment, right there on hospital bed number 4, that I had just put him through hell. I felt like a monster. At our wedding I had made a promise to him that we would be an incredible team when married, and I promised him a happy life. Only two months in, and I was already dragging him down. I called a friend the next morning and got some serious help.

Most of my friends and family were shocked when I told them I wasn't going to drink anymore. I didn't seem like a stereotypical alcoholic. I was young and fun. I had a perky attitude and great blonde highlights. But I quickly met other alcoholics who were just like me, young girls who could drink men under the table, like me. Who after three beers would pick fights and have to clean up the wreckage in the morning. Like me, once they started drinking, they couldn't stop.

I started to get better, little by little. My family noticed a difference, and that's when they stopped asking me if I was a "real alcoholic." There were no more horrible nights alone in my apartment, or hospital visits, and Allen noticed his stomach stopped clenching when I said I was coming home late.

I learned what it felt like to wake up without feeling guilty about what I had done the night before and without the trepidation of having to apologize to someone I had offended with a uncouth comment or accidentally kicked during a drunken dance-off. I started to have more confidence in myself.

And still, even after sobriety, even after the cobwebs cleared, I still wasn't ready to talk about my diagnosis. I could focus on only one life-changing event at a time. It took me about two years of being sober before I could address that part of my medical reality.

BIG BOOBS, BIGGER DECISIONS

I have been a victim of assault, and I have been harassed and teased for my breasts and body. And like every single woman in the world, it seems, I was attacked. This was three months into college; it was a huge violation of privacy, it completely rocked my world, and it took years to recover.

Men have told me what they think about my body without being asked. It's infuriating because I don't care if it is considered a compliment in your pea-size penis brain. It is none of your business. I was not put on this earth for you to comment about my body.

To avoid rude comments, I covered up. If I didn't think I was skinny enough, I covered up. I wanted to live my life as a happy woman confident about her body, but it was easier to be buried. Like a sexual burrito. My story isn't unique: Every woman I have met has trouble with some part of her body. Except the six women in the world with perfect bodies who are currently having sushi being served on their crisp stomachs.

At least my boobs were a lot of fun during sex. During sex I can let my breasts finally breathe like two fat birds escaping their cages, flapping in the wind. I want to be sexualized when I want to be. I want to be a dirty, gritty, spankable seductress when I am alone with my husband with a sound machine and iTunes radio playing. (Because in our NYC apartment, we can hear our neighbor breathing.) When we have sex, I want to feel free, and Allen is the only person I want to see me in that way. Otherwise, I keep them on lockdown, because otherwise my breasts will enter the room before I do and steal the show.

Life with Allen was fun and exciting, and it all started off with the wedding. When we got engaged, I decided that our wedding was going to save me and my anxiety. Instead of making doctors' appointments, I got to work finding the best florist and made sure we had an ice cream sundae bar for dessert.

Cancer wasn't a priority, but the size of my breasts was. It was my big day, and somehow I needed my breasts to defy gravity. I wanted an off-the-shoulder dress, and I was going to fight for it. I went to a trendy bridal shop, ready to explain my predicament. "Yeah, we know," the bored hipster attendant told me. "It will be fine." She was unimpressed. That's not the answer you want to hear when you are afraid your breast will pop off during the vows.

At every fitting I reminded them that the dress needed more support or maybe some extra boning to keep everything in the right place. I was given a rehearsed half smile and told I shouldn't stress. Her eye roll confirmed I was being *Such a Bride*. It worked. I stopped asking questions and figured I was being overdramatic for my first wedding. I wouldn't be as emotional by my third.

Two days before the wedding, I tried on my dress for my dad, and as we zipped it up the last button popped and

the dress zipper broke. SEE, LADY? MY BOOBS are going to RUIN this wedding—if I don't go to jail for ruining
you first!

I was in a straight panic and began to cry. My dad immediately called his fanciest friend, who knew a seamstress,
Michelle, who did work for beauty and drag queens. My
body fitted perfectly between the two.

Michelle applied a fishing-hook type of contraption to
secure my breasts and had it ready the next day for my wedding. I was locked and loaded and felt secure without a nip
slip or too much pain. If I could have every single item of
my clothing tailored by Michelle, I would definitely be a
nicer person.

We had a killer wedding. We danced to Belinda Carl-
isle and Nas and smashed cake into each other's faces and
did it again on our honeymoon. I was ready to start my life
being Allen's wife! My breasts were right there with me.

But more and more, I no longer wanted my breasts to
run the show. Aside from the threat to my very existence,
they also ruined perfectly good head-shot sessions. Did I
want to forever be cast in roles like Shoulder-Pad Hoarder?

Suddenly, the idea of getting a double mastectomy was
growing on me. I could be safe. I could be photographed. I
could fit in button-down shirts. Pretty soon I was Googling
reconstruction and *implants* and fantasizing about pretty little B-cup bras. But what about Allen? He knew I didn't want
the surgery—he'd heard me rail against it since the day of
my diagnosis. I would have to explain this complete 180.

Allen is careful and wary of most of my plans, like the
one where I open an armadillo sanctuary. I was good at hiding my fears from Allen. I would talk about dying of cancer
only right before bed, or right before sex or at dinner in a

fancy restaurant, or at brunch, or while he was trying to read or pee. I actually tried to hold back my crazy thoughts, and then a louder voice in my head would say, YEAH, BUT CANCER THO!? And then whatever we were doing or talking about had to be silenced.

Even though I proclaimed to the world (my family) that I would never ever have a preventative double mastectomy, I thought about it often. The process included removing all of the breast tissue down to the breast wall, because those cells had a much higher chance of becoming cancerous in my lifetime. The milk ducts, glands, and all the fatty goodness would go. Meaning I would no longer be able to breast-feed our future children.

Was I doing a bait and switch on Allen? I had already cut out alcohol, which was a staple on our dates, and now I was cutting out boobs? Had he had enough handfuls, snuggles, licks with my ginormous chest?

We sometimes talked about a possible reduction because he saw how hard they were to lug around. And I had trained him to examine any outfit I wore to make sure my boobs were in check. And he didn't mind that I would wear a bra during sex sometimes to avoid my boobs clapping for me during the act.

Would Allen be upset with a surgery that removed the option to breast-feed our children? Once he got really upset when I gave our plants cheap fertilizer because he thought I was pumping them with plant steroids. Would he be more upset our kids would never receive "the world's most perfect food," according to *those mothers* with *those blogs*? We would have to feed our children formula, like the plants. Will formula make our kids sugar addicts with

ADD? Was I going to be a terrible mother before I was even pregnant?

Also, Allen would have to end his love affair with my breasts. He got to enjoy them for only five years. The first time he saw them, he said for a moment he almost believed in God. I was taking away one of the featured amenities he signed on for. I had plenty of questions and fears running through my head, like:

- Would I miss my breasts?
- What if this was all a huge mistake because I was gambling with fate and my body?
- Would Allen think less of me because my boobs would be fake?
- Would I look like a stereotypical '80s stripper, and if so should I maybe get a perm?
- Would the new breasts feel rigid or plastic?
- Since Allen married me with big knockers, had they been false advertising?
- Would Allen look at me differently after seeing my body go through surgery, and would my scars make him uncomfortable?
- If I can't breast-feed, would I be shamed by hip Brooklyn moms?
- Would feeding my kids formula make them sad, fat babies? If I did have a fat, sad baby, should I start an Instagram account for him now? He should probably have a signature hat, right?

But I was so unhappy, and scared, and I was obsessing about death. The head shots were just the final straw.

Something had to change. I had been in this boobie prison for too many years. If I finally got rid of these things, would I also lose my fears of dying of cancer?

The fantasy grew. I would never need to have another painful mammogram; I wouldn't worry that my life would follow in my father's family's footsteps. OMG YES! I wanted that relief.

Why wait? Why can't I take that control back now? Was I going to spend the rest of my life, living for an age when I felt I could make strong decisions? A time after kids, when my body was my own? Why was that fifty-five?

It was time to take back my body. It was time to have the mastectomy. I just had to tell my husband, and I had to have his support.

So I was going to have to work really hard at this. I had to be smart and not too emotional and careful with how I phrased everything, or he might talk me out of it, like when he nixed my armadillo-farm enterprise. I had my work cut out for me. That meant it was time for sushi.

SERIOUS SUSHI

I created this Sushi Scene because I knew this extreme procedure would be a hard sell. But I wanted this surgery, and I didn't want to back down. I was ready for a long, complicated discussion, but ultimately this was my body, my future, and my choice. But my choice influenced his life. If I stuff him with sushi, will he notice I am going to change our lives forever? How much sushi is required?

I wish I was a girl who could meditate through big life decisions and sit quietly in silence as the answers to all my questions are slowly revealed. That's not a style I can ever live up to. In stressful situations, I like to know food will quickly be served. That's why I love having major life discussions in restaurants. You can't get too crazy because you are in public, though it's acceptable to cry a little, and after there is always dessert. There is always an understood time limit to the whole event, and throughout it the waiter comes by to give you little breaks. It can be awkward, but it's always worth it—just like the dentist.

We loved Sakura. It was the best place to tell Allen about my life-changing decision. It was our favorite sushi restaurant, we knew the owners, and he loved the one-dollar sake. We met the owners when they first opened and became friendly with them over the years. I babysat their kids, and they would take us to awesome secret restaurants in Flushing with incredible lotus-leaf dim sum. It's the perfect place for me to set my plan, park my coo, and persuade him.

So that's why I strategically chose to tell Allen about my decision for a double mastectomy there. I really didn't know what he'd say, how he'd react. If I supplied him with enough seaweed salad, maybe he wouldn't care that I wanted to remove his favorite body parts?

Allen was telling me about his day, I think. My heart was pounding, and I was planning his reaction, my reaction, the waiter's reaction! And amping myself up for his slew of questions that were sure to follow.

I couldn't take the pressure any longer, and before our appetizer had a chance to be delivered, I took a deep breath and announced, "You might totally freak out and hate what I am about to say, but I think I want to have a mastectomy." That's how I did it! Just threw him into the icy water without any warning. And I kept going! I pushed forward and told him all my fears, feelings, and that I was inspired by Angelina Jolie. If the hottest woman in the world didn't care if her boobs were fake, why should I? That I hated my body during my head shots and I was sick of covering up my breasts.

I went on. I told him I would find the best doctors on the planet and make sure everything would be covered by insurance. That I felt like I was waiting for my life to start after the surgery, that I would do this in the most thorough way possible. That I wanted to get the surgery now before we had children because I was rushing having children so I could get breast-feeding done and out of the way.

I just kept going. I told him how I was sick of suffocating my sexuality and that I could have more control over my body with this surgery. That I could design my own breast size!

The waiter interrupted and Allen inhaled. I ordered the moon roll, dragon roll, and a large unsweetened green iced tea, and then I kept going. I explained that I wanted the relief of not having to worry about getting breast cancer, and I wanted that relief to start as soon as possible. Then I think we both exhaled. Before I started crying like a retired soap star, I let him speak:

"Okay, whatever you want to do."

Wait—what?

"Yeah, I mean if you want to do it, I support you. It's your body."

"Don't you want me to breast-feed?"

"I wasn't. I turned out fine."

"Me neither!"

"Great. Then who cares?!"

"Oh my God, this is insane."

Insane! Wasn't he going to mourn in his miso over my soon-to-be-gone-forever G cup? Wasn't he going to cite the dangers of submitting to a knife?

"It will be fine," he said. And he told me that he wanted what I wanted—my happiness and a long life together.

Apparently, I talked about my BRCA diagnosis and cancer fears all the time, and he was feeling the pressure right alongside me. "Yeah, and saying we have to hurry up and have kids so you don't die of cancer isn't exactly a turn-on," Allen confessed.

Touché, husband! That does sound like a shitty thing to keep telling your lover. I was so far up my own ass filled with fear that I didn't even notice I was dragging him through all of this with me.

That sushi meal went on record as being the fastest, easiest life decision Allen and I have ever made together. Picking a vacuum was much harder. Allen explained he was there to support me, but ultimately it wasn't about his approval. It was my body. SHIT, THIS GUY IS GOOD.

Allen blew my mind. He was okay with me doing such a huge surgery, which only made it more real and means that it's actually happening. We kept eating, and he kept listening to me as I dumped out all of my thoughts. And HOLY CRAP, you know what happened? The scariest thing ever suddenly wasn't so scary.

It was incredible, the weight was lifted. I was going to get a surgery that would be life changing and end my fears of breast cancer. Allen finally wouldn't feel pressured to have children before we were ready. And I would finally have the breasts I always wanted.

So we ordered dessert. And the next day, I called Sloan Kettering.

HOW TO SHOCK YOUR THERAPIST

My favorite thing to ask my therapist is "Does this make me crazy?" It's a good question. I love therapy because there is someone who is qualified to tell you if your thoughts are cracked out or not. Most offices have a degree or two hanging on the wall, and there's always a full box of Kleenex within arm's reach. It's a very safe feeling, the way a mental institution is safe.

My favorite therapist was Susan, whom I saw for a year in college. Her office was in a bad neighborhood outside campus, but the risk was worth it. Susan was a quiet woman with short white hair and a slight lisp. She had a long tan-leather Chesterfield sofa, worn in with hours of worry, self-expression, and tears. I fitted right in. I compare each new therapist to Susan, and every session starts out the same: asking if *[insert current anxiety]* makes me crazy, to see if they'd respond as soothingly as Susan had.

It is hard to find the right therapist in New York City. The market is flooded with smart, helpful people, all of whom don't take insurance. The ones who do usually require me to take six trains and a bus and then cross a river, just to find they only treat pets. I finally found a new therapist (let's call her *Not Susan*), and she was fine. Her office was near my job, she took insurance, and she wore deodorant.

I was seeing her because of my anxiety and stress with life/work/cancer/waking up on time. You name it, I had anxiety about it. She was always fifteen minutes late to each appointment, but I didn't require much from *Not Susan*. We discussed the usual: my career fears, my money fears, my sober fears, and my baby-planning fears. But today was different. Today I was going to talk to her about having a preventative double mastectomy. And all I needed was for her to say, *You're not crazy.*

This was going to be perfect. I would have a certified *okay* from a mental health professional. As a result, all my conversations about it would be easier. Explaining this huge decision to my family, friends, and occasional gas-station attendant would now be a breeze with *Not Susan's* stamp of approval. My family didn't always trust my judgment, since most decisions were solely based on 3:00 a.m. Google binges.

Not Susan's office was not remarkable. It was always a little too hot, there was only one small window—too high to see anything interesting out of—and zero artwork. It was the size of most New York City offices and most Texas closets. At first it was my little retreat, but I started to get sick of it. The uncomfortable burnt-orange IKEA chair with a nonfunctional orange pillow was no longer cute. That day she was wearing a teal skirt and orange tights. This woman loved orange.

I sat down. This time I was more clearheaded than I had been in previous sessions. I knew I wanted this surgery, so I sat across from her going over everything I rehearsed on the commute over: cancer followed me my whole life; I don't want to live with that fear daily; having the surgery is better when I am young because I will heal faster; my breasts are too large and have been a problem for me for too long; I've wanted a breast reduction since puberty.

Cue puberty memory:

Usher's "You Make Me Wanna . . ." is playing in the Victoria's Secret as my aunt Valia gives me a handful of silky bras I had thought only prostitutes or cool moms wore. This was a huge moment. I was a lead in my eighth grade spring musical. I won the role of the Broadway Baby, a runaway who had a solo in the middle of the show and then—you guessed it—runs away. Valia and I spent hours memorizing lines, practicing my blocking, and shopping for the perfect red lipstick.

Broadway Baby was incredibly sexy, obviously, and she needed the perfect costume to match. Valia and I decided a form-fitting black leotard with leggings was perfect for the genre and my mom's budget. But I needed a bra.

"Ooh, Caity, this one is perfect. You are going to look like such a knockout in this," Valia proudly said, holding out a jet-black padded bra.

"Um, uh, I just don't think it's right for me," I said, horribly embarrassed because I knew a real actress wouldn't be afraid of her budding sexuality. But I was. I wanted to vanish into the bright-pink striped wallpaper of the dressing room.

"Okay! Let's do this one!" she chirped.

Valia found the perfect modest bra for my performance and then took me to get a Frappuccino. I relaxed, relieved that was over but feeling better than I'd expected. I wasn't growing up too fast, and I wasn't becoming someone I was afraid to be.

I sat across from *Not Susan* and explained all the reasons I wanted the surgery. I even told her about the pressure it put on my relationship with my husband and my fears of dying of cancer. After my announcement, I took a deep breath and looked to her for her pronouncement.

I waited for her to sit back, give me the big thumbs-up, and say I was making the right decision. I was looking for validation. And maybe a hug?

Instead, she pulled out her notebook. "How is your body image today?"

Huh? Um, bad, duh. We talked about that last week, remember?

The questions kept coming, each one implying I was, in fact, crazy. Or if not crazy, then overly emotional, possibly irresponsible.

But I knew in my bones it was the right decision. Even when she stared at me blankly, giving me no response, a silent disapproval, not even a meaningless courtesy nod. I was right and she was wrong.

I was shocked that she didn't agree with me. My ears started to get warm, and I wanted to vanish into the scuffed beige walls. She listened, but I could tell she was not on board. *Not Susan* wanted to be sure I was making this important decision for the "right reasons." Of course she was—that's her job. But she didn't understand.

"Everyone on my dad's side of the family has died of cancer," I told her again. *"They all died,"* I repeated, slowly.

She wrote something down in her notebook.

"I grew up constantly looking over my shoulder. When I was little, I was convinced my sister would be diagnosed with cancer," I tried.

Still silence.

"Plus, my breasts are huge, and they aren't getting any smaller—no matter how much weight I lose."

"Have you tried to lose weight?" she asks, stone-faced.

Duh! I am a woman. Of course I have tried to lose weight! Do you want me to circle the fat?

"I was thinnest at my wedding, and they were 32E," I countered.

I wasn't backing down. It was fine if she decided I was crazy. This was my body. I was going to have this surgery, no matter what. I wasn't going to get her approval, and I was fine with that.

"What size are they now?" she queried.

Uh, she wants to know my cup size? Was this something they teach in psychology school? Exhaustedly, I pulled back my shirt to show her my actual silhouette buried under my carefully chosen layers of sweaters and scarves. "Big," I answered.

She looked. Her eyes widened. "Oh, wow! Those are quite big."

"Yeah. That's what I have been saying . . . "

"I didn't realize they were that size. Wow, you hide it really well!"

Suddenly, she was interested. "My best friend had a breast reduction and said it was the best decision of her life," she proudly reported.

Was she on horse tranquilizers? What was happening? The threat of cancer didn't move her, but my big bosom in her face got her going? Where was her diploma? What adult wears orange tights? This was *Not Susan*, and her approval no longer mattered. I was getting the surgery, and I was never coming back here again.

I said thank you and wrote my check out to her and in the memo field wrote, You're fired.[*]

---

[*]   I actually kindly said thank you and paid her fifty dollars for my copay and walked back to work.[†]

[†]   I got a one-dollar slice of pizza and then went back to work.

DOCTOR, DO YOU LIKE ME?

By way of Google, I found the doctors I would need to remove my boobs and build me a new set. I had to choose two doctors from the same hospital. One oncologist for the first half of the surgery, the mastectomy, which would remove the breast tissue. The other would be a plastic surgeon for the second half of the surgery, my reconstruction surgery.

I had no idea what I was doing when choosing a doctor. Mainly, I wanted a supersmart workhorse who was also a perfectionist but also kind and also wouldn't be bothered by my onslaught of questions. I hunted ancient message boards, medical review sites, Facebook groups, anything I could get my hands on. I read important things like which doctors have good eye contact, who made rude comments, and what doctors smelled the best.

I picked the doctors with the most comments that included "made me feel comfortable." Here were some doctors who were touted as the best in the field, but they also happened to offend patients or rush them out of appointments. I am too sensitive for that. I need a doctor who will hold my hand, go as slowly as I need, and tell me which Spice Girl I remind her of.

Once I narrowed the choices, I stalked the doctors online. As you do. I read even more interviews with them, scrolled for Twitter mentions, looking for any details to know them better.

You can scoff at my system of research, but this time it worked, because it turns out for once I actually made great choices! I fell in love with my doctors immediately: Dr. Pusic and Dr. Gemignani were both soft-spoken and sensitive to my needs. They seemed to like me, and they liked each other. They typically operated together on the same patients and had a great relationship. I had joined the Sisterhood of the Operating Pants!

Dr. Pusic, my plastic surgeon, wore a blush rose–colored lace dress and cream heels. HIGH heels. I wear heels for only about twenty minutes max at weddings until my pinkie toe threatens to break off. As far as I'm concerned, after you spend a decade of your life in medical school, you have permission to wear bunny slippers and pajamas under your lab coat.

It's a little embarrassing that her appearance made me feel safer, but it did. It was like I was in a high-end department store to purchase a bag twice my rent and not just to use the restrooms. Plus, admiring her cute shoes and wrinkle-free dress was the perfect distraction from my constant worry about how much pain I might be in after surgery. Instead of fretting about stitches, I'd think, *I bet she knows the best brunch places in Portofino, Italy. I bet she dry-cleans all her clothes. I bet she doesn't even need Spanx and never sits in traffic.* The medical instruments, sterile supplies, and scratchy gowns were drowned out by the superficial story I made up in my head.

Mostly, I knew she was a brilliant surgeon and specialized in this surgery. I wasn't ever worried about her ability to do great work. I was afraid of how I would respond to surgery and how my body would be forever changed. She knew the perfect type of implant for my body type and examined my breasts with respect and a seriousness that made me feel I was in the right place. She knew exactly what she was doing, and she was ready to get to work.

I hoped my surgery would be her most favorite surgery of all time. I wanted her to think *This girl is fun* as she sewed up my left boob.

The day I met Dr. Gemignani, my oncologist, I immediately wanted to be her favorite patient too. I'd have bought her affections if I could. I can't treat her to a weekend away at my ski chalet in Vail, but I can make her laugh about my nipples. And did we laugh about nipples. Being a brilliant oncologist is exhausting, but this woman looks like she just had a blowout.

Dr. Gemignani had an open and generous demeanor. She had met girls like me—that is, anxious balls of emotions—and she knew how to work with a wacko. I never felt like I was taking up too much of her time or she was rushing off to another patient.

I was one of the younger patients she had come across, and she respectfully wanted to know why I wanted this extreme procedure. I explained my decisions based on my family history, my anxiety with the future, not feeling comfortable with my large breasts, and the pressures BRCA was putting on my life and my marriage. She listened to it all and said she admired how meticulously I thought about this decision and felt confident that I was ready for this surgery.

It was amazing to be around these two smart, sophisticated women. They had it all, and I wanted to soak it up. Maybe during the surgery, their cool-girl power would slowly seep out of their hands and into my body, just enough for a small cool-girl transfusion into my bloodstream. (So far I haven't noticed a change, but this could be one of those slow-moving transference instances.)

I'm not a shallow person, but I also love looking at pretty people, because it's fun. These women were gorgeous. How did they have time to wax their eyebrows while also keeping up with a busy surgical schedule? I bet they can afford to laser all of the hair off of their bodies.

I wanted to hang out with my doctors, eat expensive tapas with them, and find out how much Dr. Pusic spent on *those shoes*. These were women I admired, respected, and wanted to vacation upstate with. I really wanted them to like me and laugh at my jokes. I also wanted them to keep me alive.

Both women were calm and confident, and I couldn't wait to let them get to work on my sad sacks. They were self-assured and made me feel as though my surgery would be just another boring day at the office. That sounded good to me. I want zero excitement while they had my body opened up on a table.

Some people (a-holes) might say that surgeons are given too much glory or have a God complex. That's exactly what I want in a surgeon! I'm INTO them feeling like God, because until this moment, no one has made any alterations on my body *since God*. I'm pro having reverential confidence in anyone cutting open my body. And I will take two badass, chill-AF women for my surgery. Please.

CAITY CHATS HER FACE OFF— LIKE, A LOT

I like to think of myself as a private person, but that is just a comforting lie. One month before my surgery I couldn't keep anything to myself. Every human I came in contact during this time heard my entire story, whether they wanted to or not. For example, one day, I walked into Sephora and was greeted by a sales associate. "Hello, how are we doing today?"

"Hi! How much for this concealer brush? I am getting a preventive double mastectomy because I have the BRCA gene—not breast cancer, so don't worry! And I won't be able to move my arms for who knows how long. I need to stock up now—because I don't know when I will be back able to ride the subway again." I smiled and waited for a hug.

"Thirty-five dollars," she said.

I didn't think I was being incredibly self-involved; I was just really involved with the self-inflicted impending doom. It was all I could think about. Every time I saw a friend or had anyone ask me how I was, I would say, *Well, I*

am having this huge surgery . . . blah blah . . . terrified . . .
blah . . . needles and blood . . . blah . . . doctors cutting me
open . . . blah blah . . . cancer . . . But it's elective surgery. I
was very fun. Most people just wanted to tell me their problems or see if I had any hot goss. Hot goss is always the most
popular topic.

I didn't know exactly how I would feel or react after
surgery, which made me go insane—so I decided to talk
about it constantly, which made me go insane. I would rid-
dle off facts about surgery like when my brother was trying
to explain Yu-Gi-Oh! The more words I used to describe
the process, the more control I had over the situation—that
was what I kept telling myself.

It would be cool if I was one of those private, demure
women who are subtle with feelings. Not this lady. I just
told my dog walker about my postnasal drip—it's a big drip.
I was always encouraged to be a classy woman who uses
economy of words. As this book proves, that's not happening anytime soon. I bet classy girls don't cry almost exclu-
sively on public transport.

I repeated my fears over and over. I was more predict-
able than a plastic plant. I had the same record on repeat.
There were cancer organizations and support groups that
work with women to help them avoid this exact problem—
obsessive, nattering fear—but I didn't know about them at
the time. And besides, anything officially cancer related
made me recoil like a hot flame. I didn't have breast cancer, and I didn't want to associate with cancer groups. So I
avoided it all, entirely.

No matter how many well-intentioned people reminded
me, "You don't have to do it," that's not what I wanted to

hear. What I wanted was to speed everything up and get the whole process over with.

Meanwhile, I had a good time finding new things to worry about. Here are some of the things I imagined could go wrong during surgery:

- One boob becomes reattached to my back.
- I lose the ability to love.
- My doctor's heirloom wedding ring gets lost inside my chest and I have to explain to her that it now belongs to me.
- They open me up during surgery and a small family of tiny aliens emerges, seeking diplomatic immunity.

Combined with these logical fears, I am the world's worst patient. I hate doctors' offices. I hate blood tests. I hate scratchy gowns. I hate the color beige. But I might get cancer, so I have to be a patient, and not just any patient— one who elects to have incredibly invasive surgery. This gives me more things to hate:

- I hate the BRCA test.
- I hate MRIs.
- I hate the term *presurgical testing*.
- I hate checkups.
- I hate that under eye concealer.

Once I got out of my self-pitying bubble, I went to the most useful place for information, YouTube. I hunted for women like me, women who were electing to have preventative mastectomies. There are 6 million videos of chinchillas in top hats but almost nothing about my situation.

Women had shared plenty about breast cancer mastectomies, and I even found one woman who had a breast cancer scare and chose to have the surgery to avoid future brushes with death; she had a horrible experience and spent the next three years correcting her first surgery. Her story was heartbreaking and uncomfortable, so I watched every single video she posted.

Still, she didn't deter me from getting the surgery. I had a good feeling that my body was young and healthy, and my doctors were practically bored by mastectomy surgeries because they had done so many. I would be fine. What she did do was clarify just how alone I was in this experience— where were the other people who were my age, with my diagnosis, getting preventative surgeries? They were definitely not on YouTube.

I knew I couldn't be the only young woman considering this choice. But I might just be the only one willing to talk about it! (A lot, apparently.) Hmmm . . .

And that's how *Screw You Cancer*, the documentary, was born. When I first came up with the idea of telling the world about my life with BRCA, I considered blogging— easy, fast, cheap, and I could post some of my before photos (*not* the ones with the blazer)! But then I had a better idea: I could take my story to the world via a camera. I could tape myself in brief videos, and I could talk to viewers before and after each doctor appointment.

I contacted my friend Megan, who blogged for *Glamour*, and ran the idea by her. I figured maybe *Glamour* would help me get my project off the ground by featuring some itty-bitty-titty blog posts about me. Megan liked my idea, so we sent a Hail Mary e-mail to the magazine editors.

And guess what? They liked the idea! They asked me to come in right away and meet with Cindi Leive—the freaking editor in chief of *Glamour*! No pressure, Brodnick. I couldn't believe it. I'd be talking to women who helped shape what it was to be "cool," and I was going to *tell them about my boobs*.

How did this happen? I was not Glamorous. The last item of clothing I bought was a pair of leggings from Amazon.com. What if they thought I was ridiculous? What if my cardigan was so last season? Do people still wear cardigans? I had no idea what I was doing.

The day of our meeting, I fussed with my outfit up until the very moment I exited the elevator and was escorted into the offices of *Glamour*. Then I was brought to a small office with colorful pictures of French bulldogs on the walls, and suddenly I let all of my nervousness fade away—I felt right at home. That day, *Glamour* and I became best friends.

The editors sat with me and the bulldogs, and we talked about my ideas. I told them I hoped they'd let me post a series of blogs following my surgical journey. I tried to appear relaxed and mature, like someone who has her shit together, but of course I just overshared like I always do. (It's always a gamble when you ask me, "What's new?" Get ready to hear about the fart that woke me up last night.)

Luckily, they wanted to hear my story from beginning to end—so that's what they got. Every single agonizing, embarrassing detail. I told them about my dying family, my diagnosis, my decision-making process, how I felt about surgery. I told them all of it.

Then they told me *their* idea. Not only did they want to feature me on their home page, but they also loved my idea of filming my progress and wanted to create a documentary about me and my journey with BRCA. The editors explained how it would work: They would have a camera crew follow me over the coming weeks and months, capturing my visits, surgeries, and recoveries. Then they would create a documentary series in six segments, or episodes, that would air on the *Glamour* website.

I took it all in, my mind reeling. I was a little speechless, I think, but of course I said yes. I mean, duh. I was going to talk about my boobs to tons of strangers, but I had good material and not just the kind that was overflowing out of my scoop-neck T-shirt. Plus, I figured all of this was going to be in my comedy act, so I might as well try out my material with a camera crew first.

We got started right away—*Screw You Cancer* would be happening in real time, and we were only twenty-five days before the surgery. There was zero time to reflect—we had to start rolling ASAP. Filming for the episodes would begin immediately, and the footage would be edited and posted within a week of filming so that viewers could experience my life alongside me, without delay. We sprang into action.

It was a probably a good thing that there was no time to pause—I might have second-guessed the whole tell-it-all, boobs-in-the-news deal. As an actress, brutal honesty wasn't new for me, but typically when I perform I have some distance from the story I'm portraying. I'm perfectly happy to stand on a stage and talk about the time I pooped my pants in the apartment of one of the richest twenty-three-year-olds in Manhattan, but I usually need a little time and space to properly process the destruction I caused before telling the world about it.

The advice from my favorite storytelling teacher, Margot Leitman, is to tell a story from your past only if you are over it. You have to be past all the muck and drama and therapy to do justice to your story. This allows you to better comment on your life experience and not turn the performance into a venting session. No one wants an audience to demand a fifty-dollar copay after your set.

Not this time! I was about to get real with my oversharing, and hopefully the viewers wouldn't be too uncomfortable. *Screw You Cancer* was happening *now*, and it was *real*. This wasn't that story from school when I stayed in character as a runaway teen a little too long after rehearsal and my director had to send people to come look for me. A film crew was hired and tasked with getting up-close and personal with me, and Time and Space were not on our staff. Luckily, I figured, I would be heavily medicated during most of it.

Mostly, though, I was honored. I wanted to help women by sharing my experience, and I was excited. I could connect with people on a large scale and create a community for women like me. And I'd be doing all of that with *Glamour*, which meant my story would be living inside a happy, pink, bubbly website, next to articles telling you what hair color you should pick based on your face shape. I hoped that having the hot-pink sway of *Glamour* would gently introduce my story to women who were as timid as I was. When there are fun lip-gloss colors to look at in the

margin, the cancer story in the center isn't as overwhelming. It was happening!

Screw You Cancer helped me, too. It made me get up
in the morning and brush my teeth, because I had a job
to do, which was to show other women they weren't alone.
I would imagine all the young women who were in my
same position, feeling paralyzed and afraid to take action.
I wanted to create a conversation with women who might
have been too uncomfortable otherwise. I also wanted to
get a free subscription to *Glamour* for life, which will happen any day now. I can feel it.

I met the director, Cathryne, and producer, Grant, for
the first time at an outdoor café, where my friend had a
wedding reception five years earlier. She is now divorced
and we don't speak anymore, but the soup is still good.

Cathryne told me a little about herself, and two sen-
tences in, I was in love. She wore a flowy turquoise-blue
shirt (my mom's favorite color) that looked elegant and relaxed and spoke to me, saying she was exactly who I wanted
to spend the next six weeks with. The meeting was terrific,
and I looked forward to spending hours of intimate honesty (including nudity) with Cathryne. But then she said
she wanted to meet my parents and talk to my family. I, of
course, got anxious all over again.

Why did they have to meet my parents? They had already been through so much—they didn't choose for me
to have this surgery, and they certainly didn't choose to
have a documentary crew follow them around during one
of the most stressful times in their lives. I was ready to jump
around and play goalie guarding my parents' feelings. I
should protect my parents from this crazy plan, right?

Instead, I ran the idea by my parents, and they quickly agreed. Still, I obsessively texted my mom, telling her over and over that she didn't have to talk about anything she didn't want to and that I supported her if she wanted to opt out of the entire project. She had my blessing to throw a shit storm and flee to Target if things got too emotional.

The day of the meeting came, and of course I had worried for nothing. The second my parents met Cathryne and the crew, they all fell in love, the same way I had. Cathryne must have been wearing turquoise that day too, because my parents felt as safe with the team as I did. They talked about me, and cancer, and their lives, and when they were done, they exchanged cell phone numbers and hugs. They even made a plan for my parents to spend some time in front of the camera, talking about their experience with cancer. When it was over, they waved good-bye like long-lost friends.

The gang was all set. We were going to tell this boob story, and we were going to do it together.

DIRTY-DANCING WASPS

Right before my mastectomy, I started having some super-ficial concerns. Like, this surgery felt slightly dangerous. Also, recovery was going to be difficult, with a whole six weeks before I could work out. Being bedridden does have its perks: Most people will bring you cake. But I was worried about the lack of exercise and how my body would react to the surgery. What if I hated my body after the surgery? What if my horrible coping habits (Munchies and Media) made me gain a lot of weight?

I had no control over what was going to happen during the surgery or any idea how I would recover, but I could go on a trendy preemptive diet. I quit sugar and told my family and friends to skip the cake. I would stick to healthy smoothies and balanced meals.

Now, I knew I had an unhealthy relationship with diets, but this time I was *just* going to cut out all sugar and make my family abide by all my wishes. Very low-key, nothing ag-gressive or drastic. I should know the difference because I have tried every single fad and type of diet out there. I can't get enough. I love to read what morning elixir celebrities drink before award shows and what voodoo magic they used to lose fifty pounds of baby weight overnight.

I figured I would lose some weight by cutting out sugar because my favorite food group is dessert. Given the chance, I will reason with you why I can eat an ice cream sundae for breakfast, lunch, and dinner. I stand by it: Breakfast should include dessert!

Dieting made me feel like I was doing *something*. Maybe I should have focused on strength training and detoxing from coffee and unhealthy foods in general. But I couldn't think that clearly. I was scared, and I had to toss sugar overboard to keep this ship afloat.

The diet went fine at first. I lost ten pounds! Then we had a family vacation with my mother's side of the family right before my surgery, to spend time together and to say bye-bye to the boobs. We all went—parents, grandparents, aunts, uncles, and cousins—to just spend some time relaxing before the inevitable medical storm rolled in. We trekked to a resort in the West Virginia mountains where my family had gone since my mother was nine. It looked like the resort from *Dirty Dancing*, but for WASPs.

It also happened to be the most delicious place in the world. The food was all home cooked, with a lot of love and butter. Of course I broke my diet. I can't pass up homemade moose-tracks ice cream every night. Don't you remember Chapter 3, where I confessed I am not a hero? My no-sugar diet died. I had no control over the upcoming surgery, and now I had no control over my sweet tooth.

I thought I was an expert dieter! I can't help but try every trendy diet that comes with a world of possibilities. Some make you lose weight immediately, some make you sick for days, and some make your feet orange. Each with their own charms and glaring WARNING signs. My parents tried to instill the importance of healthy eating and regular exercise, but that's superboring. Drinking purple juice that makes my burps smell like licorice and regret is way more exciting! I heard that when Paula Abdul did it for her nineteenth comeback, it involved something with deconstructed chia-pudding cups.

I am a sucker, and I am well aware that the diet industry is my reliable used-car salesman. Any intelligent doctor will tell you a healthy diet and lifestyle give your body the best chance against disease. Any crazy girl will invest in a juice cleanse as an excuse to lose thirteen pounds.

Plenty of people want to lose a few pounds, but it takes a real sicko who hopes to be put on a strict anticancer diet to require her to stop eating ice cream. Yeah, I'm a grade-A sicko. The more dramatic the diet, the better, to try to keep me from my natural diet: waffles-'n-ice-cream-in-bed-on-the-reg.

I'm fascinated by women who willingly just eat a little bit and can "take it or leave it." Excuse me—leave it? Why would you hurt its feelings like that? Food has feelings, right? I want to be someone who can stop herself at one serving. How luxurious. I will even settle for someone who pays attention to being full. Both are exciting novelties I'd love to experience.

My favorite diets are the easy kind, like acai berries. You might toss them in a salad, or buy a lifetime supply from Costco and eat them by the handful while scrolling through Twitter. Either way, you too can be a part of the new movement. In fact, I have purchased trash magazines in hopes they will bully me into some new relationship with my body that doesn't involve stuffing it with doughnuts at three in the morning. I haven't found it yet.

For this reason, I love diet infomercials. I love how hopeful they are and how exciting the Afters are. The reveal in the second act of the infomercial is the best part. I wish I could wake up every morning as a reveal, to a live studio audience, applauding the transformation I achieved while I was sleeping.

I love that in twenty-two short minutes, you are convinced how this product will change your life, bring families together, and, more important, make you hotter than ever before. Most infomercials star a forty-five-year-old man who "has a better body now compared to my twenties!" Well, duh. You were drunk, roaming the streets of New York City, looking for free hot dogs. But with only thirteen and a half minutes a day, I too can have a life worth celebrating. And sure, anyone can afford sixty-five easy payments of $34.99. All of that is doable!

My first purchase was the Ab Slide, then Windsor Pilates, then the Tracy Anderson Method, a few makeup products here and there. And everyone and their au pair had Proactive.

Right before my wedding, when I still had my huge old knockers, I was cast in an infomercial as a weight-loss Before. I was thrilled! I was going to be in a commercial, my dream come true.

Commercial "Before" testimonials are always classic, no matter what the product is: Life is hard, the job is a burden, and time with the family is limited. If only they had enough money/friends/lashes/mineral powder, life would finally be worth living. Guess what? All those worries can be solved with a hair brush that can also whisk eggs. And you *must* try this organic foot cream so you can finally wear sandals because we all know your coarse, sandy feet are keeping you from true love and understanding!

I had been trolling Craigslist, like the beginning to all great stories, when I saw the audition for a health commercial. In the breakdown it asked if you wanted to lose weight—*uh, yeah, always.* The suggested requirement was for people who wanted to lose fifteen to thirty pounds. I had a solid six I wanted to lose, so I applied, hoping they weren't hung up on math. For the audition process, you had to say why you wanted to lose weight more than anyone else. They were looking for confessional videos and a good sob story.

I could be amazing at this. I live for this. I DVR-ed Brazilian butt lift! I have purchased a hose that stretched up to fifty feet and immediately shrinks when it's empty, and I don't even have a garden! I was perfect.

I also like the courtship that is involved with commercials. I like that they start at the beginning, how the contestant really hates their garbage life—and how this product can be the one thing that brings them from jumping off a cliff into a rocky demise. The journeys seem fun and not like they have to try too hard to make the best decision they have ever made. Everyone wants to be sixty with a body "better than they had in high school." That's the mark of a great commercial: the actor trying to relive his or her glory years. I also like the group scenes when the models are doing their fifteenth take of lunge squats and are still smiling. Bless them.

This was even more perfect for me because I was getting married in three months and wanted my wedding dress to hold me in a little better. If I lost a little more weight, maybe my boobs would finally fit! I wasn't letting these girls betray me on My Day. I was going to get as skinny as possible to keep them under wraps. So in the audition, I told them I wanted to look perfecto for my wedding day, to feel "better than I had ever before!" Gurl, you know I aced that audition! They loved me! I was going to be "the featured bride."

The other contestants and I quickly became close; we were a little chubby family. We were told not to mention if we were actors or performers, but we all were. One divorced dad worked as a clown on weekends, one girl knew every word to Nicki Minaj's song "Spaceships," and a grandmother was classically trained in Shakespeare. We were basically theater fat camp for adults. The best part was that they would send packaged meals to all the people in the program because the Food and Drug Administration (FDA) needed some proof in order to advertise that this weight loss plan actually worked. We would record our food and send it in, week by week, abiding by the program guidelines. I wasn't hung up on truth in advertising, but I did like FREE FOOD.

The product offered a thirty-minute workout program and nutrition pamphlet. We Befores were offered fifty-minute exercise classes that followed the workout video schedule. For us, because we were so lucky, they offered two classes a day to accommodate everyone's schedules. We were encouraged to attend both if we wanted to lose a "little more weight a little faster." It wasn't mandatory or even recorded in our journals, but we knew if we didn't lose weight promptly and within the time frame, we would be CUT. We were a bunch of out-of-work actors, so it was totally worth it.

Potentially being cut motivated us to work as hard as possible because not making it to the end meant we were too fat AND too slow at losing weight, which was more horrific than sleeping next to Trump. If we didn't make the cut, we'd be sent home to cry into our remaining dried, frozen meals.

Suddenly, it was a three-month audition, and the payoff was a new body we were bullied into keeping. Because did I mention that NO ONE WAS EVER PAID? This wasn't a moneymaking deal at all. Still, if I lost weight and shrank my tremendous tatas, it would be worth it. The first month was fun, just like any other exercise class. But then the personal e-mails started, and I got a little concerned. My in-box was inundated with motivational e-mails that reminded me I "don't want to regret my wedding day" and that I "only have one honeymoon." They reminded me of my (their) goal to reach 110 pounds in the next month. I asked a few of the other contestants if they were getting these specific e-mails, but no one had.

In the middle of the program, I had to take a hiatus for my wedding. And as you already know, it was the most amazing day of my life and one I had been dreaming of since I knew how to walk. We had a gorgeous and magical day, better than we could have imagined. As for my boobs, they barely shrank. They were there, loud and proud, but I managed to contain them.

I came back from our honeymoon and had gained five luxurious, joyful pounds. I was immediately bombarded with disgust and disappointment by the infomercial team. "How could you do this after all we worked for?" one of the fitness trainers asked. *Um, I don't know. I just had the most amazing time of my life, with the love of my life, while you were home licking frozen peas. That's how?*

We still had one month left until reveal day, and the producers' encouraging e-mails got stronger. Their propaganda worked! I did "cool tricks" like other contestants by eating only spinach all day. Sometimes I went above and beyond and threw it all up, like the overachiever I am.

I quickly confessed to my mom that "it feels so good to just get all that food out of my system after I eat it." She immediately explained, "Honey, that's bulimia." No! What? Me?! That's impossible. I wasn't bulimic. I studied that in middle school! I saw that Calista Flockhart movie! I'm a feminist!

How could I be bulimic? Since I got back from my honeymoon, I threw up only every few days and twice on weekends. Go figure?

Yeah, I had become bulimic. The truth was staring directly at me from the toilet.

I contacted the infomercial producers to say I was quitting. I explained that the program was too stressful, and the pressure I felt was causing me to be bulimic. I was embarrassed and so sad that I couldn't keep it all up. They wrote back with reasons I shouldn't quit and *great advice*, like, "Just wear baggy clothes at the filming of the reveal!" That way they could hide my weight gain and still claim I weighed 110 pounds. (Um, I have been hiding under baggy clothes my whole life; they JUST thought of that.) They sealed the e-mail with my new favorite request, to "help us the way we helped you."

Hold up. Let me get my head out of the toilet to take in this message. You helped me? You bullied my ass for three months and convinced me to abuse my body. Oh, you mean the fifteen pounds I lost with dangerous eating habits and vomiting—*that's* how you helped me?

I e-mailed them back, explaining that since I was throwing up all my food, I wasn't in fact eating the meals we had been reporting in our journals to the FDA and my participation would be fraudulent. And if they continued to harass me any further, I was more than happy to report them to the FDA.

I only wish I could have said good-bye to Grandma Shakespeare and Mini Nicki Minaj. We had all stressed and sweated together to come this far, and now I had to ghost everyone.

Two months later, I got an e-mail from the head fitness director. Subject line: Your decision. She confided in me that I had made the right decision and proceeded to tell me she had battled bulimia for years and wished me good luck on my journey.

Infomercials 0, Bulimics 1.

And guess what? After all of that, my breasts were still huge. As if to say, we're ride-or-die, biatch. My boobs didn't care if I puked up frozen meals for weeks; they weren't going anywhere. My mind and body were berserk, but my breasts maintained their power pose. I could be as thin as physically possible, with breasts continuing total body domination.

MASTERS OF MEDICATION

I let go of bulimia and booze and was ready to let go of my breasts, too. But I had to make sure of one thing: I was not going to relapse as a result of the pain medication given to me during and after surgery. My sobriety is precious to me, and I am always one drink away from ruining my life and breaking my husband's heart.

I didn't want to feel high from the pain medication and seduce myself into thinking that this euphoric feeling was worth throwing everything away. I was never a pill popper, but addictions can change and evolve and I wasn't going to risk it.

Relapses happen and are equally common and deadly. I have close friends who picked up drinking after a medical procedure and lost all of the sobriety they had worked for years to keep. I couldn't handle that risk on top of my growing mountain of uncertainty. So I set up a meeting with a pain-management specialist at the hospital.

The pain team was happy to discuss my pain plan. I had to clarify I did not want any morphine or Oxycontin or any other addictive pain medication. I had to specify I wanted the lowest dose that was safe, and I assured the doctors I would adjust if needed, but I wanted to start small. They were receptive and impressed with my vigilance. If they're impressed with me, they should spend time with more recovering alcoholics.

I was confident with our new medication plan, and I went over the details with my friends and family who would be helping me after the surgeries. I drilled it into them: *I only want to take the lowest recommended doses. Got it?* I also asked Allen and my mom to record my medication so they could help me if I accidentally took a dose too soon. I was intense, but that didn't surprise anyone.

It turned out I was smart to be careful. Later, during my recovery, I would feel slightly fuzzy from the medication and immediately stop taking it. It would turn out the mediation I was given was in fact highly addictive. It might have been my hyperawareness or an act of God, but I stayed sober throughout all of my surgeries and I am forever grateful.

IF THESE WALLS COULD TALK, THEY'D VOMIT

Remember all the times I told you I'm a medical wimp? Here's evidence. I had a lot of doctor appointments before my surgery, and I trembled walking to each and every one. I was even shakier in the waiting room. I couldn't focus enough to read the stack of juicy magazines like *South Dakota Living*. The words would jump around, my dyslexia and my anxiety would make wild love, and I couldn't focus on the *buffalo-berry doggie-treat recipe*.

Sitting in the waiting room, I thought of all the cool projects I could be working on instead of this mastectomy. I wanted to write a one-woman character show about a fairy who has to earn money by working at an office, but she can't figure out how to use the computer so she writes on the screen with a permanent marker. I know, GOLD. Later she sits on the keyboard for a butt massage. I can't help that I'm a genius.

I told my doctors about my anxieties, and they advised me to meditate, and that made it even worse. I wish I could breathe through my stress, but instead I would think about all the simple ways I could die during this process. Nothing flashy—just some microscopic cell bacteria would fall from the ceiling into my chest while I was cut open and then ravage my body from the inside out. I would first lose my sense of smell, then my fingernails, and so tragically lose the ability to scratch-n-sniff.

Worry was the center of my world, and everything else was orbiting in an orderly panicked manner. I eventually forced myself to stare at my phone and watch mindless Internet videos to distract myself from my own brain. I was one of those wild kids at the Italian bistro who would become muzzled over a good *SpongeBob SquarePants* episode on Mom's iPad.

The waiting room at the cancer center is designed to be friendly and welcoming. It has light colors and clean lines. But it is still a cancer center's waiting room, and I couldn't shake the feelings away, no matter how soothing the carpet design. As I sat and tried not to hyperventilate, other patients entered, looking equally worried and anxious, waiting for treatments or results or answers. No one wanted to be there, but there we were, trying not to feed off each other's angst.

I might never have gone back after the first time if it wasn't for the friendly receptionist, the hot-chocolate machine, and the free graham crackers. Other patients and I would stand around making our double-chocolate French-vanilla lattes and agree this machine was our light at the end of the appointment. Every checkup I had, I almost canceled the day before. Then I'd think, *graham crackers*.

My siblings also loathe shots. When my sister was two, she punched my mom in the face when she was struggling to get out of her vaccinations. And then when my brother was little, he punched my mom in the arm! I never took a swing, but I did need to be heavily bribed. My mother refuses to attend any medical appointments since we have become adults. One day I told all this to an uninterested nurse, and she said I'd better toughen up if I wanted to be a mother because when you are pregnant, you are constantly getting stuck with a needle. Nice nurse. Real nice. To be fair, she was very pregnant and very over my dainty veins.

Besides, I have a solution to all this. More doctors' offices should pump in cake-batter perfume through the air vents. Wouldn't it be wonderful if the waiting rooms smelled like birthday cake and looked like a toy store, with vitamin gummy dispensers on the walls? Did I just revert to a child in my waiting-room fantasy? Uh huh, hunny. Each chair could have its own private TV, like an airplane, so you could block out your own reality and watch *Rugrats*.

They should also provide you with a goody bag of spa samples after each visit. Because you actually showed up, you deserve to be pampered! You can now have the rest of the day off and luxuriate in a collagen-boosting face mask.

There should also be a Lisa Frank glitter mural of a puppy dancing inside a dolphin's mouth who's riding in a sports car made of rainbows. There should be a small conveyer belt of magazines, like a modern sushi bar, delivering you magazines from the other side of the room so you don't need to get up.

There should be a raffle for gift cards—if your name is picked while you are waiting, you get fifty dollars to Dave & Busters.

It's the best way to get friends and family to come with you to appointments, because who doesn't love a raffle? And the energy won't just be focused on the impending doom that will come when they call your name.

That is my dream waiting room. Also, free money falls from the ceiling and Idris Elba's hotter cousin whom we have never met because he is working on preserving wildlife in Australia is your doctor. I warned you, this is a dream.

THANK YOU. COME AGAIN.

I HAVE ANXIETY AND SO CAN YOU!

The term *presurgical testing* sucks. Why do they need me to go through testing *before*? Is it a test to see if I can handle surgery? How about I just tell you I can? *How many blood tests and free-boob hangs would I need to endure?*

For my last presurgical appointment, I made Allen take off work to come with me. This time, I didn't want to end up vomiting and fainting alone. I wanted him to hold my hand and to keep me calm. Of course, as soon as we arrived, I was irritated at my husband for being so calm and for my sweaty palms. In sickness, and in health, and in anxiety?

The nurse came into the exam room, and I promptly told her I was nervous and hated having my blood drawn, but also I loved her sweater. "Oh, we don't have to do any of that, hon. I am just checking your blood pressure, height, and weight and going over what to expect on the day of surgery," she said with a warm smile.

That's all? Then why did they call it "testing"? I cried a few tiny tears of relief. This was going to be the easiest appointment I had ever been to. Allen was right to not be worried. We finished the entire appointment in ten minutes, and I left with my little packet of instructions for surgery day.

Things I literally could have done instead of worrying:

- learn how to use the Marcel curling iron
- pluck my toe hair
- throw out that jar of jalapeño jelly stuck to the bottom of my fridge
- bake a layered rainbow cake
- embroider a tablecloth
- collect rare Dutch postage stamps
- start a charity
- breed illegal hedgehogs
- invent a pet-friendly computer
- admit "I don't love *Friends*"
- close a charity
- learn about anal bleaching
- dust
- write a spec script for *Legally Blonde 3: Baby, Bondage, and Blonde Blessings*
- finally make that baby blanket for my friend's eight-year-old
- learn about monarch butterflies
- e-mail my grandpa and ask how his watch-repair hobby is going
- visit the Kimchi Field Museum in Seoul, Korea
- wash my delicates
- create a travel blog for rodents

Sometimes all it takes is a no-needles day to make me happy.

SUPERCHILL COLD FEET

The closer the day of surgery came, the more amped the *Screw You Cancer* team became. Whenever we met, I told them I wanted to be as transparent as possible. I wanted *Screw You Cancer* to show all the gritty details everyone was too precious to show.

I told them I didn't want to be cloaked in the romantic pink wash so often given to breast cancer survivors. I know women who feel it trivialized their cancer experience and romanticized the very difficult process of treatment. I have been told that the angelic halo around breast cancer survival can feel more annoying than helpful—the idea that if you stick a pink ribbon on something, it will help cure cancer makes them feel diminished to a logo. What other disease has become trendy and cute? Zero.

I did not want *Screw You Cancer* to upset cancer patients by getting it wrong. So I clarified my vision with the camera team over and over, drilling us all until I was sure everyone was clear about our plan, like an Olympic gymnastics coach. Because soon it was all systems go for a full reveal, and I was pumped. That is, until the day of the surgery.

The day came. As we knew it would. (I thought about putting "bilateral prophylactic mastectomy" on the calendar, but it didn't fit, so I just wrote, "OH Shiiiiiiiit Suuuuuurrrrggggggeryyyy"—which also didn't really fit.) The morning dawned, and off we went to the hospital— me, Allen, my parents, and the documentary camera crew, who was highly caffeinated and ready to capture every gruesome moment.

As soon as the camera crew arrived at my apartment, an icy sensation I recognized as panic washed over me. *Bye-bye control. It's been fun.* Suddenly, I wanted the cameras GONE. Did I really think this was a good idea, to have them film me in the most vulnerable and disgusting moments of my life? I might puke on the nurse; I might punch Allen in the face just to feel alive. Were we really going to preserve those shining moments on film?

I turned to my producer and started the process of chickening out. "Maybe you could shut off the cameras for a little while, . . . " I stuttered. "Maybe you could come back . . . a little later?"

The producer took my freak-out in stride. He wanted to confirm I changed my decision and kindly reminded me that this is what I had wanted from the beginning and that I might regret not including this part of the process. He was right. This was why I created *Screw You Cancer*, for these exact moments.

Just like that, I came to my senses. YES, I did want to cover it all. It was incredibly uncomfortable, but what else was new? I wanted to take the viewer with me during the entire scary process. Not just leave them guessing with a bunch of before-and-after shots. I reminded myself that if my experience could help make another girl feel any ounce of comfort, it was totally worth it. We started our journey to the hospital and I was a mess, but I was a mess with the cameras rolling.

As we walked to the surgery center, I stared at the other people on the street who were going to work, living their normal lives, while I was going to have an operation that would change my life forever.

I wasn't allowed to eat anything before surgery and I was too nervous to pee, so there wasn't anything to do once we arrived but put on the hospital robe and paper underwear and sit on the hospital bed while I waited for the doctors to wheel me to the operating room. I spent some time admiring the hospital socks. They have grippers on both sides—supersafe! But that's all I liked.

They came for me almost immediately. I guess I'd expected a long wait and maybe another round of tests; I wasn't prepared at all. I had to say my good-byes and started to get weepy and jittery again.

Then a gentle nurse brought me to a pleasant holding area, and I waited to be taken into the operating room. A small curtain separated me from other women, braver women who were cutting out cancer and who had been through chemotherapy. My healthy body and I felt guilty. At least I was allowed to have Allen with me, and I kissed his face more times than I can count.

Dr. Gemignani and Dr. Pusic came to see me. The only question I could think of was "Will I be in a lot of pain?" *Yes, of course there will be pain, silly girl! You aren't waiting in line at the bank.* But I was just stalling for time. They were okay with that. They explained there would be some pain, but I would have ample amounts of medication and I would be kept comfortable.

Then the anesthesiologist came in to meet with me. He told me about the drugs he'd be using to keep me asleep, but I didn't really listen. I would have let him hit me over the head with a frying pan. I just wanted to be comatose. I didn't want to know what was happening or feel my feet or know fear.

(Pro tip: Don't tell your anesthesiologist you are a co-median. He will ask you to tell a joke. He won't think the one about a drunk cat is funny, but he will let you know his band performs all over Staten Island. He will ask if you are famous—you aren't as famous as he would like—and he will then tell you his friends said he should be a standup because he would really kill. He will also tell you he lives in New Jersey and commutes to Staten Island for band prac-tice, and you will want to stab yourself with any nearby nee-dle for immediate relief.)

It was finally time to go. This was it. The surgical team wheeled me into the operating room, and I scanned the room as if I were searching for escape routes. At the same time, I was thinking, why am I still awake? I don't want to see this.

The room was kind of gorgeous, with an all-white theme, and if you could make one adjustment, you would maybe replace the floors with a subway-tile Carrara marble. Then I thought of all the blood that would stain it, and then I thought of my blood. Also I wondered, what if I pee myself during surgery? Will I have to send the nurses gift baskets, with a little card? "Sorry I peed on your floral Danskos."

I knew at least my surgeons were confident and relaxed. I didn't have time to pretape a motivational video, reminding them to keep focused and that their work is valued. They refused my offer to hire a live deejay.

I would have appreciated virtual-reality goggles so Angelina Jolie could give me the thumbs-up as I went under. Obviously, they can't get the real Angelina—that's crazy— but they could hook me up with a high-res hologram pep talk. With a little motion capture, I could choose to have a pep talk in a French café or on a private yacht circling Turks and Caicos.

She would say, "You are the most fascinating person I have ever met— and trust me, I am a hologram!" I would laugh and laugh, and then she would tell me to relax and that she will be by my side when I wake up. And then I would wake up. The fantasy would be ruined, but I would always have that time in Reykjavik with Angie.

I lay on a warm bed and was met with friendly faces and couldn't wait to be knocked out. Which I soon was.

DID ALLEN JUST DITCH ME FOR MARGARITAS?

The surgery itself was uneventful for me, though with these big babies, my doctors were kept busy. My breast tissue from both breasts was removed, and that involved cutting through the skin to get to the tissue that makes up the breast, and cutting through the skin means severing innumerable nerves in the skin. In the healing process, these nerves, as well as the little blood vessels and channels that carry lymph fluid to clear bacteria in the system, have to mend and regrow. My skin was also pulled and my muscles were adjusted, so everything felt very tight immediately after surgery. The doctor also removed my nipples. I don't have too many details about this surgery because I was asleep for all of it. I just know my doctors were confident that they knew what they were doing.

Waking up from surgery in the recovery room, I felt very nauseous. Immediately, I surged into irrational panic mode. I was positive Allen had taken the chance while I was under general anesthesia to have a torrid love affair with a nurse and had flown to Italy for lattes. Now they were laughing over my hospital bed as they sipped flat-whites. Turns out that was just a medication-induced hallu-cination, but I wasn't convinced.

"Where is ALLEN?" I tried to scream, but I was barely whispering.

"He's right here. He's been here all night by your side," my mom assured me.

"Are you sure?"

"Yes, Cait! He never left! He's currently rubbing your feet."

Hmmm . . . Likely story. I was giving him side-eye, which because I was heavily medicated was the only face I was capable of making.

Turns out Allen had been a saint, waiting patiently with my parents and rushing all over the hospital making sure my family and the camera crew were comfortable. I was so grateful that he was the man I married, and then I threw up a little. I had to be given multiple antinausea medications because whatever they typically prescribed didn't work. (I ain't typical.) And then I fell back asleep.

That next morning, I felt a little better. I was strong enough to meet with a physical therapist, who seemed per-fectly nice until she asked me to sit up and do small arm exercises so she could check my range of motion.

Was she drunk? I just woke up, and she wanted me to move my arms? I am practically learning how to breathe again, and I'm supposed to roll my shoulders back? It didn't help that she was young and superhot. How did I know she didn't just try to steal my husband from me by booking a last-minute cruise that offered unlimited mai tais? Back off, hot lady. I have finally stopped dry heaving and I still feel blurry, but I will take you down. For your own good, please leave the room. She finally did, and I promptly ate applesauce and passed out.

I was able to leave the hospital of hot doctors later that evening. No need to linger in the hospital—there was apparently a line of patients waiting for my spot so they could be cracked open and sewn up again, too. I could barely walk, but I wanted to be home and in my own bed, so I was motivated. Every few steps I took, I felt nauseous and exhausted. I finally got into a cab and was supported by pillows that my mom brilliantly thought to bring. The cab driver was terrified. Suddenly, his day was going to involve a woman looking half dead groaning in the backseat, but he did his best to drive as quickly as possible and gently dispose of me at the curb before I could throw up on his pleather. When I was finally home, I was exhausted and fell immediately asleep.

Allen cracked a few beers and brought out the good liquor and celebrated my successful surgery with the family and the crew. He was incredibly relieved and needed to celebrate. I attempted a small "woo" before I conked back out.

The next few days, it hurt to take a deep breath. It hurt to lift my arms up more than a few inches, and going to the bathroom was an event. Worst of all, it hurt to laugh. Belly laughs are how I cope with most things. I was forced to murmur *ha* like a smirking German music teacher. But I was in my bed, surrounded by my friends, family, and a documentary film crew. Five pounds of tissue was taken from my body. Even though I couldn't move, I felt total relief.

It was over. The surgery that I was so terrified of was now behind me. I had one thing to do: heal.

PRETTY LITTLE SEWER PERSON

At twenty-eight I thought I would be waking up at four in the afternoon after epic weekends in the Hamptons, not waking up after surgery with two surgical drains dangling out of my body. Drains were inserted on the sides of my breasts and were kept in place with small stitches. My breasts were numb, so it was not uncomfortable in the slightest. However, I was hyperaware I had two tubes draining fluid out of me and treated them with the utmost respect. What if I accidentally pulled on them in the middle of the night? Would they come to life like jellyfish arms and strangle me in my sleep?

The medical team had explained to me that I would have drains for a week or so. The drains would eliminate any excess fluid collected in the body, which I would want, because with too much fluid, I could develop an infection or fluid pockets. This makes a lot of sense, but also "multiple drains" makes me sound like a sewer. Most people have excess fluid after surgery, and I definitely did because my body was used to hydrating a whole lot of tissue that no longer existed. Now that the fluid was no longer necessary, my body had to adjust, and that could take some time.

Meanwhile, the compression bra they had me wear kept my body from developing fluid pockets. The compression bra was supersexy. There's nothing like a Velcro harness to keep the spark alive. Okay, so it wasn't the prettiest picture, but it held the drains in place, so I never had to worry about a jellyfish arm flying off on its own.

The worst part was "milking the drains." That's right, that's what it's called, *milking them*—you know, like a cow? At this point after surgery, I felt like a cow, so I was ready to fully commit. I had to slowly slide my fingers from the top of the drain (attached to my breast) down to the bottom, where it is connected to a little pod that then collects the fluid. Then the fluid was emptied out of the collection pod, and the amount was measured, recorded, and monitored. This way the nurses and the cruel gods above could track my progress. A slow decline in fluid would be a good sign of steady healing. The color of my fluid would also get lighter as time went on.

Have you puked yet? No? Good! Just me then! I was convinced I would faint the very first time I gave this a whirl, but it was actually easier than I'd expected. It helped that I felt nothing, thanks to all of the nerves in my chest being removed.

The drains became manageable, but I became stressed about sleep. I would have to sleep on my back until I recovered, but I am a stomach sleeper, and I have been since I was born. SIDS risks be dammed, this baby needs her naps! I love sleeping on my stomach with my right leg bent and high on my side and my left leg stretched straight. I like to feel the mattress on my stomach and try to nestle into it as much as possible.

I wasn't able to do that while my body recovered. I had to sleep on my back in a stationary position. Otherwise, I might knock or bump my chest and create a huge mess of my stitches. Precautions were taken against this dire threat. I slept propped up on a pillow, with two additional pillows on each side of me.

During the days, my favorite place to pass out was on my couch. It created the perfect Me sandwich, between the backrest on one side and extra pillows on the other. If I needed anything, I'd yell, "Allen! Bring me the juice!" I eventually learned to sleep on my back, thanks to the pain meds that lulled me into my new habits.

Staying put in one spot is essential, and while I liked the sofa, some women like to sleep in a recliner chair. One friend of mine even rented a medical bed. She fancy.

At night, I opted for the bed. Allen and I sleep in a full-size bed, not even a queen, because I like to sleep close to him. I couldn't cuddle up against him until I was fully healed, and he probably suffocated a few times under the mountain of pillows I created, but he was at least close enough to hold my hand.

After surgery all I wanted to do was sleep, and all I was doing was sleeping. I was groggy and uncomfortable, so the best state for me to be was unconscious, like my nephews at the end of all our Christmas parties.

DIY BOOBS

If you ever want to feel like an *Austin Powers* Fembot, you should have a double-mastectomy-with-spacers combo deal. Or just buy the costume online. Whichever is easier!

I know, because during the double mastectomy, after my oncologist left the operating table, my plastic surgeon took over and turned me into a cyborg. The plastic surgeon inserted bilateral breast-tissue expanders—spacers—that had been prefilled with a small amount of saline under each of my pectoral muscles. Instead of waking up flat-chested, I'd have slightly filled spacers that created a small A-cup. This felt simultaneously comforting and alien.

I understood that the spacers were used to gently widen a space behind my chest muscles to make room for the new implants. But having my body parts pulled apart like I was a rotisserie chicken is not how I thought this would go down. I thought they could just pop an implant in there, like the time they gave a guy calf-muscle implants on MTV's *True Life: I Want the Perfect Body*. Sadly, MTV is still where I get most of my plastic-surgery knowledge.

The spacers, and then later my implants, were placed behind the pectoral muscles because without the breast tissue, there wouldn't be much other than skin covering the implant. A little bit of side muscle is also used to keep the implant in place. "You don't want your implants sliding down your chest," my doctor casually mentioned. Um, no, you're right. I don't want that. I'll take one muscle bra, please. Every two weeks, I'd have to return to the plastic surgeon's office, where my spacers would be slowly inflated with additional saline until they were large enough to be replaced with permanent implants. This process might take a few months as we waited for my body to adjust to each new expansion.

When I first heard this, I almost fainted (my power move). Then Dr. Pusic explained that she was creating "a little cocoon" for the implant to live in. She had me at "cocoon"! That sounded adorable. I felt immediately better. Clearly, this wasn't her first rodeo—she was an expert at breast reconstruction and calming crazy-lady nerves. I felt like a beautiful butterfly, soon to have perfect butterfly boobies!

The spacers were comfortable enough. Each one had a small circular metal port. The nurse located that port using a medical magnet. You know, more robot stuff. When it was found, they marked me with a Sharpie marker. I've used Sharpie markers on numerous protest signs, so this part was relatable. She then inserted a long needle/medical syringe/nightmare into the metal port to fill my spacer with saline solution, slowly expanding my implant. I would see my breast rise as if I were giving chest birth to a POD-BABY ROBOT-ALIEN SPACE CREATURE. She would

expand my spacer with about 60 ccs of saline solution—
equal to about a quarter cup of saltwater—at each visit.

There was no pain because my chest was still numb
from the mastectomy surgery, but there was some tightness.
I was still on a low dose of pain meds because the surgery
was only one week earlier. When I felt a slight twinge of
nerves during the process, it was considered a good sign. It
meant that they were growing back.

The expansion process was easy, but looking at that
needle was enough to make me want to *Exorcist* puke right
on my nurse. It wasn't painful, but I was squeamish. I stead-
ied myself and made it through, plus Allen, sainted man
that he is, came with me to each appointment so I could
squeeze his hand until it was over.

Immediately after being expanded, my chest felt very
tight and a little sore. The nurse described it as "if you
had a good chest workout." The reference was lost on me.
Sometimes the pressure felt more like a fat baby fell asleep
on my chest for a few hours. Other times it felt like I was
wearing a really tight sports bra. With some ibuprofen, I
was totally fine, except for the constant fear that the spacers would somehow be filled with too much solution and I
would detonate all over the examination room. Preventing
sudden bodily combustion became my top priority.

Luckily, because my body was healthy and my skin considered "young," I responded very quickly to the gradual
fills. My skin stretched smoothly, and my muscles would
adjust to the new size easily, with only some tightness. I left
the office each time with a few Sharpie marks and a new
cup size. It's a preteen girl's dream: bigger boobies before
bedtime!

Still, I am not a patient person, and at first I was disappointed that it would take a few months to prep my body for their new and improved boobs. I get that I can't have Michelle Obama arms by imagining myself at the gym, but I wasn't liking the idea of enduring this blow-up procedure over and over again. I thought it would help to leave the doctor's office and join New York foot traffic—maybe I could feel a little more normal. But I was slower than a tourist in Times Square. I walked home thinking, "Does anyone on this street know what I just went through?!" I held my hands in front of me walking down crowded streets. Hey, SLOW DOWN! I have highly explosive packages that could bust all over my face! Be nice to me! Buy me a coffee! At least take a picture of me in front of Bubba Gump Shrimp!

When my big bongos were gone, my body felt like it was on vacation. This smaller chest felt liberating. I felt like an Eastern European model or one of the confident girls in middle school, both of which I've envied as an adult. My little bumps were wrapped happily in their new home: a medical bra. Plus, soon the coolest part of this entire experience would finally start! And it is: I got to choose my breast size!

Actually, the coolest part is not dying of cancer. But designing your own boobs is still some badass fun for a DIY-obsessed person like me. I never liked to be expanded, but at each visit I felt a thrill, knowing that perky, proportionate boobies, hand selected by yours truly (and my doctors) would soon take their place.

Finally, after five appointments, I persuaded Dr. Pusic that my placeholder boobs had reached the correct size. She had hoped to go slightly larger, but I had pined for small boobies since eighth grade and I wasn't giving up on my dreams now. I loved how my small spacers fitted perfectly in all my clothes and never upstaged me. I had a major case of giant-tata PTSD. *No more uncomfortable inflations for this girl. Bye, big boobs. See you—never.*

My doctor tried to tell me that most women who choose their implants wish they had chosen larger ones after the swelling went down. But I wasn't having it. I loved the size of my future boobs! They were perfect: large enough to be seen in silhouette but small enough that they wouldn't enter any rooms before I did. Finally, my upper body would look closer to a Russian ballerina and less like a Russian nesting doll. I was ready.

SUPERMAN'S SUPPORT

Caregiving is not a peach of a job. You want to help, but there's not much you can do. After my surgery, I was vulnerable, and my family and friends rallied around, taking care of me in a thousand and one ways. I am especially thankful to these selfless caregivers of mine, because I know that very few people have the massive, loving support I did. In retrospect, I was spoiled. Friends would sit around me in bed and humor me as I worked on perfecting my Kawaii nail-design manicures, using their fingers and toes for practice. In advance of my recovery I had ordered twenty dollars' worth of nail decorations from China, and that's a shit ton of nail decals. I was very excited. I watched nail tutorials in languages I didn't understand, and I purchased Hello Kitty nail stickers and "fake" pearl decals. Friends with full-time jobs would come over after work and let my drugged-out ass attach as many rhinestones on their fingernails as would fit.

When they went home, I experimented on myself: I like my pinkie fingers to look like they have been dunked in glitter and stickers. Medication-induced blurry vision wasn't going to stop me! I tried hard to stick as few as I could onto skin, and I might have swallowed some glitter—no one can be sure. The distraction was a gift. For a few minutes, I wasn't worried about my drains or if my scars were healing properly. I could just focus on that little sticker of the puppy with glasses and superglue it onto my left thumb.

I also relied on my friends to let me live vicariously through their normal, everyday, boob-drain-free lives. I needed to hear what the outside world was like, and I forced them to tell me every mundane detail of their day-to-day lives. Maybe it was the pain medication, but I actually *wanted* to hear about the bitchy boss who might be secretly sleeping with Jacob in the mail department and the roommate who washes his underwear in the kitchen sink and the cable guy who confessed he writes angry letters to Nickelodeon for canceling *All That*.

But it wasn't all just nail glue and YouTube tutorials. Here were some of the amazing things my friends and family did for me:

- My cousin Julia drove up from Maryland with her sweet husband, Matt, and a blue IKEA bag filled with romantic-comedy DVDs and books for me and craft beers for Allen.
- My aunt Cathy, my mother's sister, *whom I haven't mentioned yet because she is alive*, is a brilliant artist who believes in the healing powers of creativity. Right after college I was going through a bad breakup, so she and I took a pottery class together. My pinch pot sucked, but at least I wasn't crying for forty-five minutes at a stretch. Cathy sent me

art supplies I could use without leaving my bed, and I made some really great friendship bracelets out of cobalt-blue and canary-yellow thread for a girl with drug-induced double vision.

- My friend Leah bought an entire refrigerator of organic healthy foods from Trader Joe's. She then made a vegan cashew cheesecake pie, which tastes much better than it sounds.

- My neighbor Heather called regularly to ask how I was doing. Heather was fighting thyroid cancer, and she had her surgery at the same time I did. I felt guilty that while I was healing, she was getting radiation treatments. She was amazing—not only was Heather upbeat about her heroic fight, but after her treatment she went hiking in Peru! Like whaaaat??!

- My closest friends Adriana and Lauren really stepped up their A game. Adriana called when I was still in the hospital, to ask how I was feeling. "I smell," I said. The next day, she brought me a variety pack of perfume. Then she let me do her nails, even though I was high on Dilaudid. She gets me; she knows what heals my soul, and it comes in a small bottle of colored polymer prettiness. When I sound sad, she will ask, "Do you want me to come over and you can do my nails?"

- Lauren came over and shared her cheer with me and Allen. Lauren and I became sober around the same time, and when she reached her first year of sobriety, I burst into tears because I was so proud of her. She's a generous girl, and if you go out to dinner with her, she will also share her fries with you, which is the best example of friendship I know of.

More things my friends did for me that I didn't realize I needed:

- brought me ice cream
- helped me put on my shirt
- gave me their Hulu-account password
- braided my hair
- sent me pictures of their dogs taking a bath

Admittedly, not every single person in my life was this terrific. I had one friend tell me that during my surgery and recovery, I wasn't giving her enough attention. We are no longer friends. Shortly after, she moved to Las Vegas, so we are both happier.

Being a caregiver for someone going through a serious surgery is difficult. I know. I've tried. Once, when my friend Brenna was fighting breast cancer and having chemotherapy treatments, we met for lunch, and I was so nervous I spilled my coffee all over her croissant sandwich. I wanted to take away her pain, make her hair magically grow back, and kill every cancer cell in her body, and all I could do was crack jokes and make her food soggy. I wanted to be comforting and reach out to her; instead, I spilled my anxiety all over her lap.

I think I was especially nervous because I felt guilty. I had a successful surgery and was on the mend, while she was still suffering. I know my sister, McKenzie, was riddled with guilt, too. I was the sister who had the gene, and she was the lucky one without it. We had grown up as equals, but now our bodies felt very different. Still, no one can love you more than a sister, and that made everything okay. When we were little, McKenzie and I shared a bedroom, and I would wake her up at night to talk to her or climb into her bed because I was scared or bored or both. This time, she was in my bed, comforting and calming me.

She was really good at taking care of me. She was sensitive and quiet and treated me like a princess. It was like we were kids again, but this time I wasn't forcing her be my servant. This time, she wanted to tend to me out of her own free will! She brought me exactly what I needed—she always did—which was dark-chocolate ice cream with brownie bites. My spoon would bend against the stiff, solid ice cream, we would laugh, and everything would feel better.

More things my sister did:

- sang me to sleep
- listened while I described my dream home and which kitchen backsplash would be the most interesting and least distracting
- helped me sit up and get out of bed
- helped me dye my hair pink
- rubbed my hands
- made me watch Kelly Clarkson music videos

My brother was in college and couldn't come visit, but he sent me comforting text messages and called between studying macaque social structures and winning in beer pong! He and his friends would sit and watch *Screw You Cancer* then call me with cheers and support.

Other than Allen, most of my care came from my mom. My dad was there before and after the surgery but had to return to Maryland to run his physical therapy practice, but my mom came to help for three whole weeks. Our apartment didn't have enough room for her to stay with us, so she rented an Airbnb a mile away. We were really happy she was so close by, but she could have done with a few less penis portraits over her bed. The bedroom came complete with black satin sheets, a leopard-print blanket, and a black light.

Despite the beauty of her lodgings, she would come to my house to help with *every single thing, every day.* She fed me and cleaned me, and she also made me leave the house. "Let's just take one little walk around the block," my mom would say.

"I don't know," I'd say.

Then she'd give me a *look*, that powerful Mom look that hypnotizes me into doing whatever she wishes, and I'd get out of bed.

The first day, that's about as far as I got. It was four days after surgery, and I was NOT READY. That short conversation exhausted me. How was I supposed to go outside into all that fresh air? How could she expect actual physical movement from me? I had just started feeling comfortable leaving my bed and walking to the bathroom on my own.

But my mother ignored me and put on my socks and shoes, like when I was in preschool. I was not amused, like when I was in preschool. Why was she making me do this? Did she really want me to be outside walking in filthy New

York streets alongside fire hydrants dripping with dog pee? I was perfectly happy turning into a bed person; my body was starting to become one with the mattress. Why muck with natural evolution? I would live the rest of my life in this bed. It would be easier for everyone; they would know where to find me.

That cruel woman made me leave my cave of pillows and expose myself to sixty-five ferocious degrees of crisp New York City fall air. Didn't she understand that strangers would be running by on their way to wherever, willy-nilly? What if someone touched me or knocked into me? I should have carried a neon JUST OUT OF THE HOSPITAL sign. Also I might fall apart—we didn't even discuss that yet! She just opened the front door, and my eyes cried out in pain at all that natural light.

Going outside wasn't even enough for her. Once we reached the sidewalk, she wanted me to walk around the block like some kind of American Hero. Who did she think I was, Kerri Strug? I reminded her that this was dangerous. What if my legs gave up on me? They had been off-duty for a while.

But as we stumble-walked a few paces, there was a moment of thrilling excitement. The moment was brief but fresh, a delirious awareness that one day I'd rejoin the world, ready to take on each day with independence and vigor.

Then I felt nauseous. My body was moving and working in a new way and didn't like it one bit. Nausea is my body's way of saying, "Time to give up, Captain, and take this ship back home." Which I would have done if my mom hadn't been steering me ahead like a wobbly toddler.

Walking helped, even though I wasn't a fan. I had developed a superadorable case of Stockholm syndrome with my bed and pillows. I wanted to stay put in my bedroom, where nothing could hurt me and I wouldn't have to experience anything but Chinese takeout and *I Love Lucy*. But every time I left my house, I felt stronger and healthier and my breathing improved.

During the walk, I would pass all the local characters: the woman who kisses my dog on the lips, the shoe repairman who always asks for a hug, the old lady who cuts children's heads out of photographs. All of them were continuing with their lives as if nothing changed. No one was worried about me—and it was pretty fantastic. I wasn't special. I was just a human trying to survive like everyone else. I was just another slow walker passing the deli on the corner filled with MTA workers and firemen. The world outside wasn't ending, even if it felt like mine was. *Nothing remarkable about me*, I thought. And that's when I started to recover.

Here are some more things my mom did for me:

- washed my laundry
- washed my dishes
- washed my body
- gave me a head massage and brushed my hair
- bought me a scented candle
- milked my drains

Allen, of course, did more than anyone else ever could. He kept my spirits up, made me tea exactly the way I like it, and brought Fig Newtons and seltzer from the corner bodega. He fetched me juice, warmed my feet, and didn't complain when I stole all the pillows in the house. I told you he's the greatest.

Other things my husband did:

- told me I was pretty
- made me laugh
- woke me up on time to take my meds
- answered my phone when I didn't have the energy to talk
- went with me to my doctors' appointments when I was scared

Things my dad did:

- called me twice a day
- took my dog on a walk
- brought Allen his favorite cigars
- entertained my visitors when I slept
- asked my doctors important questions
- got my medication from the pharmacy
- told me how proud of me he was

I CAN'T SHOWER. NOW WHAT?

Constipation is hysterical. And guess what no one told me about life after surgery? Pain medication makes you constipated. You are welcome. There I was, after surgery—I couldn't get up, I couldn't poop, and it had been about two weeks. Oh, and we were in the middle of filming for *Screw You Cancer*, and the sound and camera guys were sitting in the next room. So everyone knows: *The girl can't go!*

It took me some time to finally have a successful number 2! I had laxatives pills, I drank laxative tea, and I bought products over the counter and tried holistic remedies from the Victorian Era. My stomach felt even more expanded than my chest. My family and camera crew were all so concerned with my inflated stomach and lack of pooping, the first time I successfully moved my bowels, the house cheered. Constipation creates intimacy.

And if that weren't embarrassing enough, I smelled. I smelled so bad I could smell myself, and that's when I knew it was bad. My friends would deny it, even though I knew they were trying to be nice because I definitely needed a good rinse with industrial soap. But after surgery

I wasn't able to get my new incisions and accompanying drains wet.

"What can we get you while you are recovering?" everyone wanted to know.

"Perfume and baby wipes" was my go-to reply.

"That's it?"

"Trust me."

I begged them for it. I knew it could be two whole weeks, maybe even more, before I could take a real shower, and I needed to assume control of my body odor, because after surgery that was just about the only thing I *could* control.

As soon as the nurse told me how long I might go without a real shower, I felt every skin cell on my body. I would have friends and family visiting me every day! How could I be a good host, smelling like a dirty subway car?

I had flashes of seventh grade gym class when everyone was using eau-de-toilet spray like Acapulco Afterthought or Seaside Escape Plan deodorant and I had no idea what was going on. All of the young sopranos in my Gospel-Show Choir were wearing Love Spell, as we belted "Go Tell It on the Mountain."

After a while, I got the body-smell-control method down to a science. Let's go over the supertools you will need in your belt if you ever smell your own funk and can't bathe:

- Fresh-smelling cleansing wipes. Any brand will do.
- Stupidly sweet–smelling body splash. It wears off in fifteen minutes. Buy it cheap, and it will make you feel like a girl again.

- Moisturizing body oil. Get the oil instead of the lotion because it will last much longer. Get the scented kind, of course.
- Dry shampoo. I loved my bottle of dry shampoo until someone in my family read the label, decided it had some weird chemicals in it, and tossed it. That was the worst moment of my recovery because that dangerous dry shampoo made my hair look amazing. Let my story be a lesson to you: If you love it, don't let anyone read the bottle. Nothing will kill you if you only use it for five days! (I think.)
- Scented candles—light 'em up! You probably can't get up and out of bed easily, so your sheets aren't going to be the freshest, and plus you might have drooled a little (a lot) on the pillow last night. Give yourself a fresh, clean scent by lighting a candle or six. My favorite scents were clean linen, fresh laundry, and happy meadows—everything that my bedroom was not. Use as many as you can without burning down the house.
- New makeup. A friend gave me some packets of MAC makeup, sealed with newness that made me feel new, too. I didn't need a purple eye-shadow compact while recovering in my bedroom, but it was an exhilarating gift. The first smacking sound of pulling out a new lip gloss wand from the tightly packed tube made me ecstatic. I reapplied so much "Loud & Lovely" gloss for those two weeks that I felt like a gainfully employed porn star. It felt great.

TITTY TITTY BANG BANG: THE SEX PART

Author's note: Dad and Grandpa, please skip to page 145.

I looooooooove sex. Allen loves sex. We really, really love sex. But I had just had my breasts removed, so sex was going to be "interesting."

I wasn't just worried sex would be different after having a huge surgery—I was terrified. What if the effort to save my life killed our sex life? I had to get back at it and prove to myself that wonderful sex wasn't going to be a memory, that we could still have a great connection and I was still a sexual woman.

Sure, my breast tissue had been scooped out and spacers inserted behind my pectoral muscle, but the other body parts were still working fine, even my libido. *Especially* my libido.

This was the closest I had ever felt to Robocop, but as soon as I started to recover, all I wanted was to feel like a sensual woman ready to please and be pleased by her partner. (Cue the 2002 hit "Cater 2U" by Destiny's Child.)

The first time I had an orgasm, I was with a guy who wasn't so into my big boobs. He was a butt guy, like a guy's guy butt guy, like liked guys' butts butt guy. But what can you do? I was in college, and he talked to me for more than fifteen minutes. Regardless of his lack of interest, I was still going to enjoy myself! And boy, did I enjoy myself. I actually saw visions—at the moment I came, I was flying though the Brazilian rain forest like a tree monkey with other tree monkeys; we were jumping from tree to tree, flying and free. And so I've been chasing that monkey ever since.

Allen is amazing in bed. (I'm bragging, but I'll stop.) He has always loved my body, and he wanted to make sure I felt adored. (Sorry, still bragging. Sorry! I'll stop.) I feel fully at ease with Allen; I can laugh, I can fart, I can knock a lamp over, and he still thinks I'm hot. I really lucked out. (Okay! I'm done now! Officially stopping.)

Despite hating my big breasts all day, every day, I felt more beautiful and accepting of my body during sex than any other time. In bed, my breasts offered my partner joy (they even clapped for him) while simultaneously making me feel feminine—they finally had a purpose. With Allen I felt sexy, beautiful, and powerful, like my childhood sex icon, the Pink Power Ranger. Would I feel the same now that they were gone?

Two weeks after my surgery, I had to find out. The only other event on my calendar was *Have Mom help you shower.* Which she did. Then it was time. Mom went back to her penis-walled Airbnb, no one was around, and the time was right. I popped a pain pill and was ready to go!

Let's be clear, though—I didn't want pity sex. I had to prove I wasn't some damsel in distress. Role play can be fun, but what I really needed was to feel like myself.

I didn't want any fumbles. I didn't want any conciliatory "It's okay—it happens" or "We'll try again soon . . . yeah, soon." I would not stand for this turning into a precious Lifetime TV moment. (But if this *does* become a Lifetime TV movie, I would like to be cast as my superhot and supersmart plastic surgeon, Dr. Andrea Pusic.) Here's how it might go:

INT. BEDROOM. DAY.
Couple with matching tans and sculpted bodies are caressing each other in crisp white sheets.

    HIM   *(Whispering in her ear)*
           You can trust me.
    HER   But can I really?
           (She turns away)
    HIM   *(Confidently)*
           I know you've been hurt before.
    HER   Yeah. . . . When I sneezed five minutes ago?
    HIM   I won't shut the door on the past.
    HER   Let it go. Pretend I'm Ronda Rousey.
    HIM   I said I liked her ONE TIME!

FADE OUT.

I was mentally detached from my body and literally detached from my breasts at this point; they were now two objects that had just been replaced with man-made placeholders. The only time I looked at them was when I replaced my bandages. Thankfully, the drains had been removed by now, but my chest was still not exactly sexy or romantic. *Please, dear God, or Buddha, or Great Goddesses above, or whoever is listening,* I'd pray silently, *please let him still think I'm sexy. Please let this work. Just please, please, make him cum-a-cum-a chameleon.*

I know this sounds a little desperate, but I think it's understandable. The brilliant Dr. Sharon L. Bober, senior psychologist and director of the Sexual Health Program at the Dana-Farber Cancer Institute, explained that "one of the real challenges that so many women experience after undergoing cancer risk–reducing surgeries is how to restart their sex lives post-surgery" and that "the key is knowing yourself and figuring out what is right for you and what works with your partner." She also recommends going slowly and having a sense of humor about it—check! Check!

When I approached Allen to tell him I was good to go, I felt like a nervous virgin in my Velcro sports bra but also like an escaped mental patient. I wanted the past two weeks not to in any way influence my sex life, so I made an attempt at seeming very chill, like someone who wears a sarong confidently. It didn't go over so well, I think. Allen is a smart human with a working brain. He is also sensitive, he had just seen his wife go through major surgery, and he was now looking at my heavily bandaged chest.

"Are you sure you want to do this?" he asked. "Are you sure you're sure?"

"Yes, I'm fine," I said, trying to sound as sexy as possible. "Hmmm."

"Look, I'm great! I told you I'm fine!" quickly abandoning any sexy attitude.

I was frustrated. I had always been capable of mixing things up in the bedroom. I wanted to jump back to where we were before surgery: music on, I'm on top, a great time was being had by all, etc. But I was off my game, awkward in my body and ancient in my movements.

But I managed to convince Allen to let me climb on top. I was ready, I assumed the position—and it felt great! That is, for about three glorious seconds before I fell over.

I had zero strength. My upper body was still healing, and my quad muscles had been napping for two weeks. But for that tiny bit of time, I was on top of the world. Well, on top of Allen's world.

We gave it another try, this time with Allen on top. As we resituated, I noticed his upper body was stronger and more sculpted than I remembered. Did he always have the chest of a Greek god, or was I *that* medicated? No one can say. Either way, Allen's body was completely perfect and precisely what I had missed. I was so excited to be back in his arms, and Allen was just as thrilled to be back in this familiar place (i.e., my vagina).

We could have taken our time enjoying the reunion, like Dr. Sharon L. Bober recommended, but let's be honest, it had been a while, so we were going to get to business. We were both *enthusiastic*, albeit a little distracted by my bandages, which did their best to be mood killers, because they were jealous, those little jerks.

We had music on, but it couldn't drown out my excessive talking. That is how I make most uncomfortable situations better: I give a play-by-play. I know, that's the least sexy form of dirty talk, but I couldn't help myself. We stayed in that position for a little while, and then I suggested doing it doggie style because, hey, I'm an overachiever. That obviously failed because I couldn't support myself, so we went for an adjusted version, one that's similar to doggie style, but one dog is lying on her stomach. I don't know the name for it, but it looks like one dog might have been hit by a car and is lying facedown but is loving her life and really into it. I was lying on soft pillows and had the time of my life. It was AMAZING.

Afterward, I was grateful. All I could think was: *He came! It still works!* And *Thank you, vagina, for being tried and true and doing your best work under pressure!* It wasn't just about the orgasm. It was as if he reached a climax of happiness, acceptance, love, and hope that our lives would go back to normal.

I finally felt feminine and sexual. I wasn't a patient. I was a sex machine/wife. For a little while, I could forget about my medication station and my arm exercises and my Velcro harness bra. Our sex life was bigger than my breasts.

Allen asked if I saw the tree monkey this time, and I didn't need to. I didn't need to have an out-of-body experience. I was happy here with a man I loved, in my new body, and I was present for every moment. And it felt better than I could have ever imagined. And then I passed out.

PREPANICS

Two months later, I was feeling stronger and more like my old self. I would have been thrilled except I was already on my way back to the hospital for another surgery. My spacers had reached the proper size, my scars were healed and waiting to be reopened, and I was ready to receive my forever boobs. My chest was all set up to welcome their new tenants!

In this surgery, my spacers would be removed and my new silicone implants would take their spots. I was eager to finish my journey and get my new baby boobies! I just wasn't ready to be in a hospital again.

I should be a pro by now. No big deal, right? But my fears were climbing up my neck and sitting on top of my eyelids. My body was running at the pace of my pounding heart. Logically, I understood what was happening—I listened to my family's comforting words, reminding me that "this is a less invasive surgery." I understood that the entire surgery would be shorter and I would heal faster. All of that made sense, and I tried to remind myself the same things, but rational knowledge was quickly drowned out by flashbacks to the surgery I just had. Waking up out of anesthesia, pain when I lifted my arms, and nausea were the only memories my brain would allow. I willed myself to let those all go, but it all felt too soon.

As you know by now, when I'm nervous I can get a little crabby, and on the way to the hospital, Allen and I argued about which way was faster to get to the Upper East Side. We had made our way there just two months ago, and of course Allen was right, but I hated all of the words that came out of his mouth just the same. I was an anxious piñata waiting to explode. (Anxious Piñata is my drag name.)

My parents, Allen, and I were a few blocks from the hospital when I couldn't take it anymore. They were all walking at a snail's pace, and I wanted to sprint, as though I could get this whole thing over with if we all just walked a lot faster. I urged my walking party to pick up the pace, but Allen thought I was being ridiculous and stuck to his meandering stroll.

I wanted to scream, but instead I just grunted like an angry wife. Luckily, my dad saw the panic in my eyes. He said, "I'll go with you! They can meet us there!" He's like a professional dad! So we speed-walked to the hospital, and I arrived in the atrium with relief. I was here, the moment was here, and I was going to have the *final surgery*. After this, I could close the book on this part of my life.

Three minutes later, Allen and my mom entered, smiling and at ease. I couldn't stand his relaxation, but I also depended on it. I wanted to smack him and then immediately kiss him for being so calm, just like in a telenovela.

An elevator ride later, we were in the waiting room again. I looked around and saw that not much had changed—everyone in the room was visibly uncomfortable, waiting for their name to be called. Some seemed sad, others scared. Not a single person in that room wanted to be there, except maybe me—I wasn't particularly happy about it, but at least I had the power to make the choice, and I had voluntarily put myself in this room with other nervous patients and plenty of Purell.

I quelled my nerves by looking around for signs of change since my last surgery. No dice—it was still just as quiet, and it smelled and looked the same. My comment cards with redesign tips were clearly ignored. There wasn't a single glitter mural.

After I checked in with the unusually sexy receptionist (maybe they did decide to hire Idris Elba's hotter, younger cousin?), I prepared to wait. I considered taking a nap and thought the doctor would appreciate that I came into the surgery refreshed. Instead, I tried to piece together conversations of the other whispering patients. I strained to hear the argument between the couple reconsidering their divorce. I silently seethed in solitary indignation with the grandpa who got a shitty deal on that dining-room furniture set. I tried to overhear the details of a guy's excuse to his mother-in-law about why he didn't go to her dog's birthday party; she was not impressed.

When they called my name, I was almost disappointed to miss out on the rest of the tales they were telling. I wanted all of these mundane details and stories packed into each person's life. I needed to be filled with thoughts and worries other than my own.

But at least I would be able to take home another pair of hospital socks.

LET'S BUILD A BETTER BOOB

My body was being made over by experts and I had no control over that particular project, so I fantasized about making over my kitchen. Design is my happy place where I romanticize home renovations. I will sit and watch hours and hours of bathroom makeovers. I might not be purchasing a home in Waco, Texas, for two thousand dollars and add an herbal barn/crystal solarium, but I did have permission to paint my rental kitchen any color I wanted. This is a HUGE win for any NYC renter. I was on a design power trip.

Before the surgeries, I had scrubbed and refinished each wood cabinet with all my might, hoping my doctors would be as detailed and obsessed with my new breasts. I removed every cabinet door, deglossed the '70s orange finish, hand sanded them down, and then restained the wood in "light oak."

I wanted to buy new countertops, but that's where Allen drew the line. We don't have the money to invest in another thing we can't take with us when we move. So I splurged and got a marble kitchen table that is only technically portable and will require four grown men to carry out. Sometimes I pet it lovingly at night and thank it for the beauty and service it provides our home.

I painted the kitchen a light pink that actually turned out to be a coral I wasn't crazy about, but I kept it because I was proud of our accomplishment and because I couldn't afford four more gallons of paint and primer.

The work I did on the kitchen reno in those last few days before my second surgery made me feel productive, and I felt an immediate helplessness when my doctors reminded me that once again, I wouldn't be very active for a few weeks after the implants. Allen would have to do everything in the home because I would take this opportunity to sleep as much as possible. I wanted to make sure he was well taken care of before I cashed in all of my room-service tokens.

During this surgery, my doctor would remove the spacers behind my pectoral muscle and replace them with my permanent silicone implants. She would make a small incision using the scar that I already had from the mastectomy and place the implants in a manner that would ensure they were as pretty as possible. I would have one drain in each breast as my body readjusted to a new set of foreign objects, and once again I would go home with a compression medical bra to limit fluid. I wouldn't be able to exercise *again* for about six weeks.

I had set up my medication station next to my bed, stocking it with a lot of laxatives and fear. There was an innocence to my first surgery; I had no idea what it would be like. Would the big, bad hospital be scary and cold? Now, going into this surgery, I knew exactly what to freak out over.

Dr. Pusic said this was normal and explained how the second reconstruction surgery can be difficult for patients because it is so familiar. She was absolutely right. I knew exactly which parts of my chest would hurt and exactly how nauseous I would feel. I knew I wouldn't be able to go to the bathroom or how I would need to swing my legs to get out of bed. I didn't even know I could become even more of an expert on my anxiety. I even surprise myself sometimes.

I was also warned that while healing from this surgery, many women push themselves too hard. They are so eager to get back to life that once their scars show signs of healing, they try running at full speed again. However, the body might not be fully healed, and activity still needs to be limited. I decided I would sit still for as long as required, maybe longer, and then even longer. I mean, after all of this effort, I didn't want to mess anything up.

In a very small way, the familiarity of the hospital was a comfort—this time, I wasn't anxiously wondering what would happen next. I had seen all this before, and any decisions that I'd needed to make had already been made.

The biggest choice had been the implants themselves. When choosing between the silicone and saline implants, I had no idea what I was doing. I was told that if the saline implants leaked, it would just be leaking saltwater and your body can naturally absorb it, but if a silicone implant leaks in your body, it is more difficult to detect. In general, if silicone leaks, it will stay right around the implant, meaning it won't go elsewhere in your body and it won't make you sick. It does, however, mean that you need to have an operation to clean out the leaked silicone and put in a new implant.

Saline was looking really good at first, but then my doctor told me that for my body, silicone would look more natural and feel more lifelike. Dr. Pusic explained that women who have silicone implants for breast reconstruction like how their breasts look and feel more than women who choose saline. That got my attention, and I gave it a lot of thought.

In the end, I couldn't make any more decisions, so I let my plastic surgeon make the call. She chose silicone implants and ordered two 450-cc silicone-filled implants, made by Natrelle and promisingly named "Smooth Round High Profile." I trusted this would provide the most normal shape. After "not dying of cancer," "looking like a normal person" was my top priority. I wanted to head into my bright and beautiful future as if nothing remarkable had happened and I had the most average chest in the world.

Some women who are keeping their same breast size choose a procedure called "direct to implant." The plastic surgeon would put their permanent implant in during their mastectomy surgery. Since I was getting an entirely new breast shape and reduction, this wouldn't work for me. I did see a friend's new breasts after she had direct-to-implant surgery. She got to keep her nipples, and her boobs looked insanely good. I've never met her husband, but I heard he is a big fan.

I had considered one other option—there's a procedure called DIEP, or deep inferior epigastric perforator-flap surgery, and it works well for many women. It provides a natural shape to the new breast by building it with the woman's own body tissue instead of silicone or saline. The tissue is mainly taken from the lower belly and surrounding areas, and it gives a very realistic and natural look to the breast.

Plus, I imagine most women appreciate the free tummy tuck. DIEP flap-reconstructed breasts feel the most natural because, well, they are.

The only difficult part for some women is the amount of scarring that takes place. Because there is so much tissue needed to re-create each new breast and form it into an appealing shape, it can leave the stomach very tight. Most women I have seen have had a large scar across the lower abdomen, similar to an extra-long cesarean scar. Their new breasts also have scars that are slightly different and larger than those you'd see after an implant surgery.

I would have been willing to consider this approach, but it wasn't something my doctor wanted. Dr. Pusic explained DIEP flap surgery takes much longer because they have to remove tissue from the tummy and then put it back in the chest area by hooking up arteries and veins. The recovery process is also longer. Getting up and moving around is much harder because your stomach is healing along with your chest. I didn't want multiple incisions—I could barely keep my breakfast down thinking of the solo set I was already getting. Plus, my doctor said I didn't have enough fat to take.

That was a revelation! For once in my life, a medical professional said I was underweight for something! The last time I was underweight, I was nine months old, and I have been trying to reach that goal weight ever since. Thank God, and please put that on my tombstone! HERE LIES CAITLIN: AT ONE POINT SHE WASN'T FAT ENOUGH. (*Note*: I later found that was not correct and that I *did* have enough fat to go around after all, but I am leaving this part in for vanity.)

My doctor also said that since I was planning to have children in the next few years, she didn't even want to touch my stomach area. The surgery would have been ideal after pregnancy, when there is typically more space for doctors to extract tissue, but before pregnancy it can make the stomach too flat to properly stretch. I would have loved her to give me Disney-princess abs, but I wanted an expandable container to cook my future babies.

She did say that there is always an option that if I wanted to one day replace my implants with my natural body tissue, I could do that later down the line. And I know that after having kids, that tummy tuck is going to look real nice. But for now that was a no-go. Plus, I was not a fan of the additional scarring. It would remind me that my body wasn't normal and I wasn't like the average person. I don't want to be precious or unique. I just don't want to die of breast cancer. So for me, seeing scars is a daily reminder.

BOOBIES GO GLOBAL

After the implants were in and I was home again, I kept myself busy watching episodes of *Screw You Cancer* and reading the outpouring of support and response to the series. It
was incredible! Three episodes had already aired, starting
with why I chose to have the surgery. The audience met my
family and Allen and heard my doctors explain the surgeries. Then they saw me waking up in the hospital and trying
not to laugh at Allen's jokes because it hurt too much.

Watching the episodes, there were moments that made
me catch my own breath, like when I ask Allen what he
thinks of my new chest, immediately after my first fill. My
insecurity and need for his approval were captured on film,
for everyone to see.

There was no turning back. My boobs were online—by
choice! I received e-mails and messages and tweets from
women all over the world. I was ready to be trolled and bullied and harassed, but instead I was shown so much love
and support, it is still unbelievable to me.

After my first few moments of cold feet, I was able to
let loose, relax, and let the camera crew film pretty much

everything—the waiting-room vigils, the bedside consultations with doctors and nurses, the many trips to the bathroom for failed attempts at pooping.

There was only one thing I didn't want the world to see. I asked the film crew and producers not to put my face and naked breasts in the same shot at once. I didn't want anyone to be able to freeze-frame me for a Brodnick-boobie screen shot.

I always felt bad for amazing actresses with images floating around online of screen shots of them topless in an art film that no longer feels as tasteful. I wanted at least an audition for any film before I subjected myself to the same. My breasts would be online not only for Google-searching women who were considering mastectomies but also for leering eyes, and I wanted to keep myself safe from online poachers and creeps. The director respected my rule and was very careful.

And then . . . Then episode 5 was released, and at minute 4:06 I am *topless in the doctor's office.* And then if you missed it, you can see it again at minute 5:30! The image includes my face and torso, all together and out in the open for the world to see. The next image is of me wincing from the sight of a huge needle inflating my spacer, with my scars all new and still raw. It's not the prettiest.

I was livid! A nip slip! Well, it would be a nip slip, if I'd had nipples already, which I didn't. How could this happen? I had one rule, and it was broken as fast as I break most diets!

I had years of experience hiding from the snooping eyes of men, and now it was ruined. My boobs—and they were still *my boobs*—were out there with my face right above

them, ready to be sexualized or fetishized or otherwise dis-
respected. I was in shock.

As I finished watching the episode, I had some strong
feelings. They started in my buzzing brain and sank in my
stomach, where I felt my anger, anxiety, and worry. Then,
just like that, my anger faded away. As fast as I break most
diets.

Just as fast as the boob scene came and went, so did
my fear. I realized it didn't actually matter if my breasts
were in the video along with my face, personalized in the
most baring-of-breasts-and-souls ways. I'd wanted to tell the
whole story, and now I had. In fact, maybe it was fate—
maybe it needed to be shown, for other girls who were at
home looking for a lifeline as they made similar decisions
about their bodies and their lives.

And if some creep wants to freeze the frame and spend
Saturday night alone with my boobies and me, then more
power to him, because he's got some special kink that must
be hard to come by. I know, I've looked.

PATIENCE UPDATE: STILL ZILCH

Two surgeries down, I'm home again, recovering again. My body was healing, I had family bustling around me, and all I could do was wait. Sitting still is hard work, and I am terrible at this kind of patience, inner peace, and acceptance. I would rather lick the floor of Guy Fieri's red convertible. I'm terrible at waiting. I am even worse when I have to wait in line, and any restaurant in New York worth your money makes you wait in line. I always get stuck in the grocery store at checkout behind a lady who needs a price check on her thirty-four cantaloupes. I hate waiting in line almost as much as my dog hates a bath: We both struggle in the beginning and then realize there is nothing we can do and submit in misery, whining and drooling until the ordeal is over.

It's hard enough for me to sit still. Now I had to just lie here and let my body heal. I tried to busy myself by Googling how to make concrete kitchen countertops and what soil is best for lemon trees. Meanwhile, my friends would stop by or send a cheerful text on their way to doing fabulous things, like writing TV shows and working on movies. Then they'd go off to their exciting lives while

I was watching another Canadian miniseries about sexy werewolves.

I felt like I was being left behind. I worried that I couldn't have kept up if I wanted to. I wasn't brave enough to do what they were doing when I *could* move my arms above my head.

It was September, which was always my favorite time of year. Before school started, we would go shopping and buy new fall clothes, and there was a new set of classes and classmates to get excited about. I loved shopping in Staples for the required calculator for Algebra 2 and at least one Backstreet Boys folder. I always needed blue and purple highlighters, even though purple was always more of a marker, and when I was in middle school, mirrors and flower magnets for my locker were a must!

I also loved September because it was my birthday. September 14 is the most beautiful day! I loved the way it looked, spelled out in curling cursive letters. I loved the shape of the soft *S* and the pointy *14*.

Caitlin Brodnick September 14 was the prettiest collection of words. Egocentric? Um, yeah, but it always meant I would have a party at school and the kids at school would have to be nice to me all day, or at least until they finished their cupcakes.

Birthdays were my happiest thing. Birthday parties always required princess dresses and we always played freeze dance, and after a good ol'-fashioned sugar overdose, there would be tears but also killer goody bags. My mother or dad would come to school, they would be in the building and pass out cupcakes, everyone would sing, and it was the best part of the year.

Here I was, turning twenty-nine years old, and my mom was still planning my birthday party! It was nine days after surgery, and it was time to celebrate. My cousin Julia and her husband, Matt, were in town, and we were still filming *Screw You Cancer.* The director desperately wanted to have a shot of me blowing out my boobie-shaped birthday cake, so we gathered everyone in the family together to share this great snapshot. I thought it was corny, probably because I had just woken up and still felt groggy. I wasn't interested in creating a memorable moment.

But that didn't stop my family! They brought in the boobie cake and sang "Happy Birthday" to me, right in my bedroom. Then my cousin yelled out, "Cait, those are your actual implants!" and everyone laughed. It was a great joke!

With the do-over cake scene complete, it was time to make my first trip to a restaurant. After my mother made me take the walk from hell around my block, I was ready to walk the single block down to the most comforting restaurant in the world, which just happens to be on our street. It was time to do our favorite family tradition: eat!

This was exciting. I had new foobies (fake boobies) and was able to leave the house to celebrate them! We walked over very slowly, but inside I was pumped. They gave us a round table in the back to fit the six of us. I was excited to show my cousins the menu and point out the homemade chestnut pasta, which is to DIE for! The crusty bread was heavenly, and even the ice water was top-notch. The waiter was about to take my family's order, and then . . .

Waves of dizziness and nausea hit me like an uncharted earthquake. I had to support myself on a chair, and I had no idea what was happening. Everything slowed down, and my neck started to sweat. My face turned white, and I felt like I was going to fall over or, worse, puke on someone's calamari.

My body turned on me. I must have pushed it too hard, too fast. It was so unfair! I was sick and fuming and so mad that I could have flipped over a table (metaphorically, because I couldn't even open a jar of peanut butter at this point). I just wanted this one moment to be fun and easy. I wanted that night to feel normal, to forget about the drains and the medications and the stitches, and allow my family to celebrate and relax. My body didn't care what I wanted.

I needed to excuse myself—fast. My mind raced. Should I head for the bathroom, or should I just go straight home? Either way, I'd have to decide fast, because this lady wasn't going to stay vertical for much longer. I quickly decided that if I was going to suffer, I wanted to do it in my own home.

I begged my family to let me walk home alone so they could all stay and enjoy a night out. Just because I was a mess didn't mean they shouldn't enjoy a well-deserved night off. I assured them that there was no reason to miss a delicious meal when they could already smell the fresh mozzarella.

Besides, I wanted to be alone. I didn't want anyone to rub my back, and I was tired of being the center of attention. I was afraid I'd lash out at my sweet, generous family who had taken loving care of me and was now worrying about me, which I was suddenly and totally sick of. I wanted to feel nauseous *privately* and not have to report every symptom. I was sick of talking about my drains, my muscle pain, *our* constipation.

I found my way to the street, cursing the surgery for ruining and taking over my life. I cursed the BRCA mutation too, while I was at it. And then I just tried not to throw up.

I shuffled down the street finally alone, still nauseous, but suddenly feeling free. My emotions were coming at me fast as I arrived at my building, relieved to be home, but the exterior metal door was too hard to push with my healing chest. That wasn't going to stop me. I turned around, backed up, and pushed the door as hard as I could with my butt. My tush had never disappointed me before, and it wasn't going to start now. I rear-ended the door as I turned the key. I had to be as delicate as possible but with as much booty force as I could muster. (I'm sure that move is already a popular dance performed regularly in a college bars.)

Finally . . . I opened the door all by myself! It felt like I had just won a championship title from the WWE. It was a bootylicious birthday miracle. My stomach was still churning as I shuffle-ran to the bathroom. But I was INDEPENDENT.

Feeling like wet garbage felt much better when no one was there to notice. Everything was quiet, and the house was mine. I could breathe easily, knowing everyone was enjoying themselves at my favorite restaurant, still able to celebrate. And even though I was only half-conscious laying on the bathroom tile floor, I was celebrating too.

A few minutes later, I carefully crawled into bed, closed my eyes, and fell asleep, feeling like a queen on her birthday.

ANGLES LIE!

Four months after my surgery, it was time to take my new boobs out and buy them presents! I was a new woman, liberated and braless. My new boobies were built behind my pectoral muscles, so they look cute and perky at all times. I am braless as you are reading this, and I haven't worn one all week. I repeat: *I never have to wear a bra.*

Before the surgery, the last time I had gone anywhere without a bra, I was seven and was obsessed with giving my Barbies supershort haircuts. When my boobs came in, there was no way they could be untethered. So this bra-free sensation was something of a revelation to me.

I love not wearing a bra! But sometimes I miss the girlie ritual, and after I healed, I wanted to buy me some hotsy-totsy bras.

Victoria's Secret has always been intimidating to me. It's like the cool girls' table, and I was an outsider. Sure, I wore bras, but they weren't fun and trendy. They had to be specially ordered online from London, because they were the only ones that offered bras for narrow backs with huge cups. I had cute bras with ample amounts of sexy lace, but it was much harder to hunt them down, and they weren't cheap. I accepted it, with bitter acceptance, like never getting a seat at the cool girls' table. BITTER ACCEPTANCE.

This time, it was different. Maybe I could be part of the club of infamous sexy angels, running around and laughing in yoga pants? The doors were open to me now, and the overpriced thongs weren't the only thing I could purchase.

I walked in and smelled the supersweet perfume I knew well. I touched every piece of satin like I did when I was little. But now I actually had the money and the power to buy whatever unrealistic piece I wanted. I looked at the shiny neon-orange-lace demi-cups with matching garter belts, touching them, lovingly aware that finally, I was one of the average-size masses, picking out an average-size bra.

A woman in all black immediately approached me. "Hi! Can I help you?" Without waiting for an answer, she began flipping through stacks of bras as she proclaimed, ever so casually, "You're probably 32D."

A 32D? Did she just say I was a 32D? Oh, no, she didn't just try to take away my hard-earned C. Not happening. I didn't just go through two surgeries and twenty-nine pints of recovery ice cream to be called a D! I had an average C-cup, lady, and the hospital bills to prove it.

"Nope. That is incorrect," I informed with a surprisingly serious expression, and I marched upstairs to the dressing rooms with bras I chose *on my own*. High and mighty on my own determination, I stood in line for a curtained hot-pink room to try on my new bras. I could hardly wait, and I wasn't going to let that oblivious woman ruin my outing. Finally, a dressing room opened up, and I entered it, ready for my transformation. And then . . .

As if no time had passed, as if I were still that teen-age girl with an ill-proportioned body and G-sized boobs that couldn't be properly contained with any bras made in America, I couldn't find a bra that fit. I tried on eighteen bras! This was not supposed to happen! I designed my per-fect breasts, and I had the scars to show for it. How could it still be this difficult to find a bra that fits?

My boobs were finally average, normal, run-of-the-mill. They were not deluxe or designer; they were off-the-rack, everyday boobies, and I just wanted a pretty bra to wear over them! Victoria, you are still so high maintenance!

I tried on all eighteen again. One bra had a cup that would cut in too much under my implant. One bra gaped too much in the front. One bra was padded and made me look like I had a huge underboob. One had a cup that was too long and went up under my armpit, and another was too small and pinched where my nipples would be if I had them.

Something wasn't right here. This was supposed to my own little infomercial moment. Where was my "After" re-veal celebration? Where was the confetti cannon? I finally asked for help.

I'd been sitting in the dressing room regrouping (read: sweating and tired) when I heard a very nice sales associate outside my curtain, trying to help a family of Italian tour-ists, a woman who was really pissed the hip-hugger panty in large wasn't on sale, and a very overwhelmed man ner-vously shopping for his girlfriend. She was sweet to each one of them, and I thought she might be kind to me, too. I flagged her down and explained my whole saga. I told her about my surgeries and comforted her when she told me about her aunt's diagnosis.

Her name was Christina, and I was right: She was one of the kindest people in the world. She asked helpful questions and gave me as much time as I needed. We looked for a bra that wasn't too tight, eliminating all underwire bras because there was no need for a supportive band, though I could buy one with an underwire and cut the wire out of the cups, so there would be no risk of getting poked by a rogue wire and not being able to feel it. We didn't want a cup that was too small and would cut into my implant or possibly rub me during the day. We also ruled out anything that was overly structured—I would need a soft cup shape that could gently mold to my body.

In the end, we picked a very comfortable T-shirt bra. This bra rested gently on my chest without any pulling or gaping. She totally understood when I told her, "Think more 'picture frame' and less 'pulley system.'"

As I tried on a new batch of bras, Christina would run back and check on me while she tended to the other shoppers and tried to aid the man with the girlfriend who was clearly relying on lingerie to save his relationship. She made me feel special and completely ordinary at the same time, which was exactly what I wanted. When it was all over, I took a few selfies and sent them to my mom, to share the exciting news.

Even with perfect woman-made boobies, the whole process took about an hour. I was ready to hand over my credit card like a trust-fund kid with a solid 401k, but the checkout line was filled with Swedish tourists and I started to get a perfume headache. So I did what all savvy women do: I went back home and ordered the bras online with a promo code.

The bra-shopping experience was just as frustrating as it ever was. As if I never had the surgery, as if my body was like it had always been. But you know what?! It also felt wonderful! I had gone through all of this surgery convinced that I would be a different woman afterward, and I wasn't; I was still me. Everything was just like it always was and totally different, too. It felt good.

OPRAH'S NIPPLES

During my mastectomy, I had to give up my nipples. Many women who have this surgery arc able to save their nipples, and they have a procedure that is appropriately called a "nipple-sparing mastectomy." Because I was receiving a reduction to my breast size as well as a mastectomy, there was too much skin to remove, and my nipple had to go. Even if they kept my nipple attached to me, after the stretching of the skin and placement of the new boobs, my nipple would be under my armpit.

Everyone agreed—let's go sans armpit nipple. Instead, my doctor would remove the nipple along with any other extra skin and then stretch the remaining skin on my chest for minimal scarring. To create a smooth shape, she pulled my skin gently away from the center of my body. I know this because I had a little hair that was in the middle of my old breast, and now its new home is on my right side.

In place of nipples, I had two small scars and one big dilemma: What to do about new nipples? I could have a new set of nipples reconstructed, which was more complicated than I'd imagined. My new breasts were selected to be unassuming and "normal," so I assumed I would have nipples to match. But it's not so simple—there are all kinds of factors to consider when designing a nipple, like the color, shape, texture, and size.

Once I was given a choice, I got to thinking. Maybe I wanted loud-and-proud areolas that really hold space for themselves, nipples that would run board meetings and stand up for injustice. Proud, brave, and brazen nipples that don't take shit.

I wanted Oprah's nipples; those are some powerful nipples. I've never actually seen them, but think of the impact those nipples have had. They have hugged presidents, reunited estranged families, and opened schools in Africa. Those are badass nipples I can get behind.

I became obsessed with nipples and wanted to see as many as possible. I looked at reconstruction photos online and vintage *Playboy* magazines. Every French fashion magazine is guaranteed to have at least six nipples per issue. I browsed some Kardashian nipples, but they all seemed a little tired. Maybe I should get grandma nipples? Something with a vintage sepia tint I could really grow into? What if I picked a pair and got sick of them after a few years, like that paint color I chose for my kitchen?

So I had a few options, and three months after my reconstruction surgery, when my breasts were fully healed, it was time to pick my nipples. I felt like a kid in a candy store! Wouldn't you? What would you choose?

Option 1: Nipple tattoo on flat skin, with 3D effects and details like veining and coloring. This can be done by your hospital or by a tattoo artist. Nipple tattoo artists are incredible; they can do almost anything. My favorite tattoo areola

I've seen was in the shape of a shamrock. The nipple itself was tattooed normally, with one real proud areola. Like all tattoos, these nipples can fade over time and might require a touch-up. But since your skin is quite numb after surgery, it isn't as painful or uncomfortable as an average tattoo.

If you choose a tattoo nipple, I recommend artist Vinny from Baltimore, because his name is Vinny and he's from Baltimore. Also, he has a great portfolio online of before-and-after nipple art. My friend Karen went in the other direction and chose to have her entire breast done with gorgeous tattooed flowers as a beautiful piece of artwork. For her, it was another opportunity to create art on a blank canvas, close to her heart.

Option 2: Nipple reconstruction with folded skin from my breast and tattoo over that for coloring. If I chose this kind of nipple, Dr. Pusic would make small incisions in the skin of my new breasts where the nipple would be. She would then gather the skin around and place a few stitches to create a raised nipple shape. This would give me a small raised bump like a nipple, but the surrounding skin would continue to lay flat. I would then have to tattoo the nipple and surrounding areola for color and detail. My areola would be flat and not raised like the nipple, but with tattooed coloring and detail, it would look as natural as possible.

I liked this option because there was some texture in the final nipple but the process wasn't invasive. Dr. Pusic said it could be done in the office and would be a simple procedure. There was a risk that the new nipple would possibly deflate as my body healed. If that did happen, she would most likely use donor tissue from another part of my body to build it back up.

Option 3: Nipple and areola reconstruction with donor tissue. This is a longer procedure where the plastic surgeon would remove skin from an inconspicuous part of my body and attach that to my breast for a raised areola and nipple. That new tissue can also be given a tattoo to make it resemble the color of natural nipples. The new nipple will always be slightly erect, and so most women choose to wear a bra to help cover up the high beams. Some women will have donor tissue taken from their groin area or under the arm, and I read somewhere that women will take it from their labia. And then I fainted.

These are all great options, but in the end, I chose none of the above. That's right. I picked "no nipple." I am living the good life, friends, carefree and nipple free! Plus, I already got a custom piece of jewelry that says #NoNipples, so in a way I already committed.

At first I worried that they'd look like Barbie's boobs. Would my once-upon-a-time buxom breasts miss their little chapeaus? But there are major perks to not having perky peaks. My breasts are still soft and round and have faint little lines where the scars are, but it is only noticeable to my critical eye. I can wear any shirt, tight or loose, and my breasts look like they are in a bra at all times.

Plus, I never have to worry about a nip slip. Accidentally flashing a tit is a thing of the past for me! I confess I was a little uncomfortable when I went to get an armpit wax and had to lift my shirt, revealing my scars and lack of nipples. I tried to explain to the Romanian aesthetician, but I only knew how to say "I love you" in Romanian. She didn't care in the slightest and didn't return my affections, but informed me I waited "toooo long" between waxes.

I was lucky to have the no-nipple option. Some women actually need to have a nipple reconstruction to help cover up additional scarring or irregularities as a result of surgery. It's a little easier for women who only have one breast removed, because the doctors can match their new nipple to the remaining one.

I wear nipple stickers on occasion, like to bachelorette parties and Thanksgiving dinner. I visited the nipple section of my hospital's gift shop and pointed to the ones I liked, and they arrived on my doorstep the next week. From prepubescents to nursing mothers, they've got every size and shape covered. I chose a light pink to match my pale, freckled body. They are small and sweet and make my tits look like a kid at Coachella. It was easier than picking out herringbone floor tiles. Plus, my silicone nipple stickers are covered by insurance!

I like the stickers I have, but there are also a few private companies who make customized nipple stickers for women. The cost is more than my gift-shop nipples, but for some women I'm sure it's worth it. I can see how someone might feel comforted by knowing she has an exact replica of her own nipples. It's also helpful for women who have one healthy nipple and want a second one to match it. The company can work with photos of your nipples, so if you have any old photos that you "accidentally took while getting out of the shower," this is the time to use them!

I use Amoena Nipples currently. They are self-adhesive silicone nipples with very nice areolas. I attach them directly to my skin, where they stay in place and feel just fine. It's all so easy that I wear them for fun. Turns out my nipple stickers love being taken to Korean barbecue and free movie screenings. The nipples came with a special cleanser, and after I wear them I wash them by hand and leave them to dry on my sink, just to freak Allen out in the middle of the night.

Sometimes I get nipple jealousy. When I see a really perfect nipple, I can't help but think—does that person know how lucky they are? And then they usually ask me to stop staring at them because it's uncomfortable.

FORCED FEELINGS

Five weeks later, I'm home in an empty, quiet house. All the Edible Arrangements had been eaten, and the flowers were starting to wilt. All of my friends had gone home. I was home alone with no upper body strength and a bag of candy.

Suddenly, I got sad, and scared. I had no energy, but I felt lazy sitting around. I was bored, but nothing interested me. I tried watching an educational documentary on hummingbirds, but I slid down a reality-TV rabbit hole instead. I overate, which I'd promised myself I wouldn't do.

Some days I'd go out for coffee, and I'd look around at everyone, thinking, *Do you know what happened to me? Do you? I couldn't move. I was terrified for months! Do you have soy?*

I felt different. And not in a fun, sexy new-haircut way. I was a step behind and a beat slower than everyone else. Which was not very glamorous and could be very lonely. I didn't want to explain my surgery to anyone because I was so sick of talking about it; simultaneously, I wanted every person to already be well versed in all of my feelings, pain, and stress. I wanted to be treated with kid gloves at all times while also being very low-key and casual.

I knew I should feel lucky and grateful, and I did. My surgeries went perfectly, and I healed better than my doctors could have expected. But I was still sad. I wanted to be happy and fresh-faced, but it was impossible. I just couldn't steer my feelings away from misery.

I wanted to stop the sadness, but I couldn't, making me even more frustrated. My brain was swimming with negativity, low confidence, fear. That took a lot out of me, so I napped. I napped everywhere, anytime I could. I would close my eyes and check out from the world. I loved sleep! Sleep gave me the feeling that I could shut out everything that made me upset. The pressure in my head would start to build, self-criticism joined in at rapid-fire, and I needed to shut out this brew of self-doubt and criticism. It was always time for a nap.

Or for a snack. I wasn't surprised that I ate my feelings after surgery; that's almost a given. I come from a long line of comfort eaters. What surprised me was how I hid from people. I stopped returning phone calls and seeing visitors, isolating myself because I didn't want to bother any friends and family with my mood. I would read their happy, supportive e-mails and respond with smiling emojis, feeling like a fraud.

I wasn't skilled enough to balance my feelings of sadness with my desire to be the world's happiest patient. I have never been good at balancing anything. You offer me a cup of coffee? I take the coffee pot and your cat.

A week after surgery, I met a "cool girl." She was real cool, as in "wearing the perfect amount of leather" cool. She worked as a personal assistant for pop stars and traveled the world. She wanted to take me out for drinks, and I wanted to go! She had great stories about glam living, and I looooove great stories about glam living. I was so excited to meet her at a swanky spot and talk to her about her adventures—but I couldn't make myself do it. I canceled and rescheduled twice, and then it was too late. She went on tour to Ibiza or someplace that requires a sarong. I stayed at home with my dog and warm blankets, knowing I couldn't live up to my expectations.

I should have made myself go and worn my impractical shoes to stomp around New York City like a pop star. I didn't. I just studied her Instagram photos, wishing I was out there with her having a virgin cosmo. I wanted to be a carefree cool girl, but I also wanted to take a third nap for the day.

I was disappointed in myself and lying to everyone else. I couldn't be honest, because if I admitted I was depressed, it would consume my life and trap me forever. That's how depression works, right? I didn't know. I also couldn't allow space for my feelings. I wanted to feel cheerful and confident and had no tolerance for anything less. But I didn't feel up to it.

This felt different from my regular moodiness. This was paralyzing in a new way. I was living a double life, and it was exhausting. I didn't have the energy or the strength to show up and be the person that I really wanted to be. Why was I doing this to myself? Was it fear? Was it PTSD? Was it perfectionism? Why couldn't I return a phone call?

I wanted to leave the house, and I couldn't. I wanted to do something fun at night, and I couldn't go. I was too afraid that if one person politely asked, "How are you?" I would unload with all of my tearful feelings and worries and pain. So I stayed home.

Meanwhile, I was no princess at home with Allen, either. I would joke about my breasts to try to lighten the situation, but if Allen said anything the least bit humorous or witty about them, it could feel like an insult. I was ready to jump down my parents' throats after a comment, even though I could have made the very same one. Joking about my body is my business, and sometimes it feels like teasing when I hear it from others. It is a very sensitive line that was constantly blurred, and I wasn't helping to make it any clearer. It's hard to see straight when your eyes are closed.

One day, a friend wrote to say she was visiting New York from Argentina, where she lives now. We were close in middle school, and now, fifteen years later, she was in the United States! She saw *Screw You Cancer* and was excited to reconnect.

What an amazing opportunity! I always wished we lived closer and thought about how we would have been the best of friends if we were given the time. She was bubbly, and I admired her great outlook on life. She was the first to teach me about spraying your bedroom blankets with perfume to make them smell lovely when you jump in. She wouldn't even be awake to enjoy them! Man, was she cool.

But the night we were supposed to meet up, I couldn't leave my apartment. I felt ill; I felt overwhelmed; I felt exhausted; I felt puffy and sad. I didn't want to be that person when we reunited, so I made my lame apologies and stayed home. She flew back to Argentina the next day, and I lost my chance.

I regret not making myself shower and meet up with her. I wish I had let myself be emotionally messy and accepted that I was still in a gray sludge of a place that lived between happy and sad.

I knew I wasn't okay.

BOOBIE BLUES

You'd think this wouldn't be such a mystery—it's not like I'd never had bouts of depression before. (If that surprises you, please return to Chapter 2, where I explain about all the death in my family and my lifelong relationship with anxiety.)

I knew that taking care of myself and taking my mental health seriously were part of my recovery. My doctors' notes all included: "Female with history of anxiety and depression." #NeverForget.

Even before I tested positive for BRCA, self-undermining feelings were always there. I could be watching a play, at a meeting, or walking my dog, and the thoughts would find me. They sit just under the surface, waiting to jump out and hijack my mental conversation.

It was hard for Allen because he was no match against my mind. Worry and fear would creep in and ruin perfectly great evenings because I couldn't stop myself from bringing it up. Except sex—sex was the only time I could say "fuck it" (literally). But we weren't having sex twenty-four hours a day (unfortunately).

My mood wasn't getting any better, and I thought it might help to move my body a little. So I took a yoga class! It was my first time stepping foot in a gym since the first surgery. I was prouder than the day I got my braces off. I called my mom on the way. "This is the first time I have worked out in nine weeks!" Never mind the fact that I got the okay from my doctors to start working out at six weeks, but you know . . . the holidays, life. Oh, and working out sucks.

But this was different. This was a new day! I was starting off easy: a gentle yoga class to get me back into the swing of movement slowly. I arrived; grabbed my water bottle, a mat, and a block; and found a good spot. The lights were dimmed, the music was soft, and it wasn't crowded. I could move my body around without being incredibly close to a stranger or worrying about hitting anyone around me.

We began with a child's pose. Awesome—I can do this. We moved to a downward dog. I didn't love putting any pressure on my pec muscles, so I did a few adjustments.

Two whole poses! I got this! Look at me! I am so peaceful and yoga-full. I am a master of my own beautiful body. Why haven't I done this sooner? This is not hard at all. I followed the poses one by one, adjusting each one to accommodate my stiff body and healing boobs.

A young male teacher stood in the middle of the room, guiding us through the poses. It didn't take him long to register that I was making a lot of adjustments. Somewhere around sun salutation, the teacher looked over me, saw my modified position, and yelled with delight, "Oh, you're pregnant!" With an excited twinkle in his eye. What? Did he—no, he didn't—yes, he did!

"NO!" I hollered. "No." Deadpan. I fixed my eyes on him. I was not gracious. I did not laugh it off or make any effort to help him recover. I just said NO. No, I was not pregnant. I might have been carrying extra pounds from overeating and underexercising, but the only babies I had inside me were silicone twins and I'd earned them and the stitches that kept them in place.

The class looked over at me. Some people were shocked. One woman was so startled, she farted. Some people were yoga-stoned and had no idea what was going on.

I like being the center of attention but not like this. If it were physically possible, I would have magically teleported myself out of the room and into my bed while immediately losing ten pounds. But I couldn't, so I didn't. I stayed in the same room and moved through to the next position, pigeon pose, which I hate because it makes no sense and because I can't do it. I wanted to kick and scream, and storm out, but I didn't. I finished the class, with a sucked-in stomach and fury in my blood.

Pregnant. I wasn't pregnant. When you have a baby, you can show the world that your body has gone through some trauma and that is why it looks the way it does. I didn't have anything to show, unless I flashed him my cool new boobie scars, which I decided wasn't appropriate.

I wish I was one of those hot supermodels who can bounce back from babies, surgery, and tabloid scandals and be in a bikini three weeks after. But that is not me. It was going to take me more time, and I had to somehow grow comfortable with it, which is not easy. I was, however, comfortable with never going to that yoga class again.

As we moved toward the last pose of the class, I wished I really was pregnant. It would be so easy. That's a formula most strangers can understand. I wanted to lie and tell them I was pregnant, after all. I'd just been joking earlier.

Ha ha ha! People would be really nice and excited for me! And maybe they'd even be impressed that I did little more than lay on the mat for the entire class! We could have had a feel-good moment and moved on.

Or I could go through my typical, truthful explanation: "I had a preventative double mastectomy to avoid getting breast cancer, similar to Angelina Jolie. You know her? She is a UN special-envoy ambassador? She's Lara Croft, Tomb Raider. Yes, she is very hot, yes, divorced from Brad Pitt. No, I don't know if she has a home in Hawaii. Anyway— the surgery she had? I did that. So I had that surgery, and now I am healing."

Instead, I said nothing. I wasn't up to teaching the entire class about my surgery. I just want to make modifications in a yoga class with a teacher who just graduated from high school and then go home.

It shouldn't matter to me what people think about my body, but in that yoga class it really mattered. I had a major life change, and my body looked like it had a major life change. I figured since I transformed my top half, my bottom half would follow. No luck. I did look out of proportion at the time, but I didn't want anyone else to remind me. I designed small breasts, and because of my surgeries I was still bloated, tired, and not in the best shape, giving me a nice three-month pregnancy pouch. I moved slowly and was still somehow sweating. I needed a moment without self-criticism, and I thought I could do it in that yoga studio.

On the way home, I fantasized about being pregnant instead of, well, whatever I was. The entire situation would have been way more fun if I was pregnant. I would be welcoming a new happy life, planning out gender-neutral nursery-room colors, and picking which milk bottles prevent gas retention.

I thought about babies and children, and that cheered me up a little. I know I sound like your mom's old hippie friend from college who makes her own kombucha, but babies are my key to happiness. Babies don't care if you are having an existential crisis or if you are stressed over your tax return. They want to play with that big red truck with the sharp edges and fall asleep in a cardboard box. They want to squish avocado in their hands because it feels good. They want to jump in that lake to see how fast your reflexes are.

If your life is falling apart, kids don't care, and it's amazing. Your focus has to be on the task at hand and nothing else: build the block tower, rock him to sleep, wipe her mouth before she smears spit-up on the velvet pillows.

I find peace with babies, so I called my most stylish friend, Nikki, who has the most stylish baby and invited me to have a picnic in the park. What do you know? It got me out of my funk! Snuggles and chubby baby legs just make me feel better.

I also went to a new doctor and worked with a few mental health professionals, because they are my favorite kind of professionals. Turns out I had depression and was putting too much pressure on myself. Huh? Ya don't say!

Once I allowed myself to admit how I was feeling, things slowly (superslowly) got easier. I was still exhausted but began my climb back to my normal life, or something like it. I just needed more time to heal physically and mentally than I budgeted. I still want to have everything figured out, but as I've proved to myself over and over again, I never will. I still get lost in the supermarket. (In fact, I'm lost right now. I'm by the yogurt—please send help.)

I had this expectation that as soon as I had perfect-looking boobs, I would suddenly be able to handle stress, diet like a master, and play competitive sports. I would no longer be the girl who sits at home and eats a family-size bag of Doritos during a Twitter war over the validity of *The Great Muppet Caper.*

I still haven't made it back to a yoga class, but I did buy a really great yoga mat. Baby steps.

SURVIVOR'S GUILT

Ideally, I would have been an actor working on the set of a cool movie that helps break stereotypes and change lives. But until then, I had to pay rent with another day job, as a receptionist at a busy law firm.

Turns out I was awesome at the job. I am great with people, I am pretty organized, and I have strong communication and multitasking skills. I am warm and friendly and was in charge of the front desk and ordering big group lunches, my exact skill set. I always made sure to have everyone's favorite cookie. I was a mini catering manager/receptionist, and I had great health insurance. Superfun!

That was all before the surgery. I was given time off to have my mastectomy and assured my office I would be back after a few weeks of recovery. One month later, I was barely able to get to work on time. Just getting there was an ordeal—I was nervous around people on the subway, worried a frantic commuting New Yorker would elbow me in my healing breast. I often arrived late to work with my hair in a messy bun, no makeup on, and still groggy.

I wanted to be that same bright-eyed and happy girl they hired, but it just wasn't the same. Coworkers who didn't know what I had been through must have thought I had a nervous breakdown. I sure looked like I did.

I wanted to tell every person I saw that I just had a life-changing surgery and I can't believe I made it into work. But I kept everything secret. I wanted to tell everyone that there are more important things in the world than their lunch order. But of course I didn't. I felt exhausted and wished I was home in bed with my husband and dog, making friendship bracelets.

I was doing much better, thanks to the therapy and Prozac, but I still felt detached from people, I felt alone, and I couldn't relate to anyone I worked with. I couldn't focus on simple tasks. I just no longer belonged. I felt as if I were looking at everything from a distant lens, a sad lens.

After my reconstruction surgery, my work started to go downhill. I had had a life-changing experience, and I didn't care if an attorney got his favorite paleo cupcake. I was distracted, fuzzy, and prone to mistakes.

I didn't want to cater to any more people. I wanted to take care of myself and my family and nothing more. I couldn't sit still and act as if nothing had happened. I felt like the meaning of life was getting lost in a stuffy, expensive office, like I was swimming in the opposite direction from the people around me. I had changed in a big way. I was also just plain sad.

My favorite thing about the job was the "Mommy Room." It was a room in the office reserved for nursing mothers. It was home to a breast pump, a computer, a recliner chair, and blackout curtains, and the temperature was always kept cool.

Since I had all of my breast tissue removed, I will never be able to breast-feed, but I loved that room. I was never disturbed while I hid, because attorneys were terrified they might see an exposed breast. The perfect threat.

I would sneak into my new sanctuary during my lunch break and lock the door behind me. I could curl up in the large recliner chair, use my coat as a blanket, and shut out the world. I would put on my headphones, set my phone alarm, and sleep as hard and fast as I could. This wasn't difficult. I can sleep anywhere—on a bus, on a plane, on a person. A true gift. The room smelled like stale breast milk, but I didn't care. This was the only way I could survive. I needed these breaks, from the people and from my racing mind, while my body was still healing. I may not have had any milk glands, but I used that room more than any other woman in the office.

I kept my experience as private as I could, but some coworkers would catch me going into the Mommy Room and roll their eyes. They thought I was hiding a secret pregnancy or just lazy. I didn't care. I pretended I was a Russian spy, impervious and exotic. (Not the spy you are thinking of, with the sexy cat suit, the other spy, the chubby one with a drowsy eye.) I was occupying enemy territory while they were on lunch break, at risk of being discovered at any moment.

A handful of coworkers knew about my secret, including one receptionist, Heather (the heroic hiker). She was diagnosed with thyroid cancer right before my surgery. While I recovered from surgery, she went through treatment. We would sit and eat gummy bears and talk about how stupid the demands of the day were and how we were happy to be alive.

I loved the solidarity—finally, I wasn't alone! But I felt like a wimp compared to her. She would leave for radiation treatments, and I would go home feeling like a fraud. I just wanted to curl up like a Popple. Remember Popples? They were fuzzy animals that could turn their insides out and transform into little bouncing balls when needed. Like a softer, cuter armadillo.

Through *Screw You Cancer*, I'd met incredible warrior cancer survivors—women who run triathlons, jump out of airplanes, have six children, jump out of airplanes with six children, and still have time to get balayage color-hair treatments. They proudly wear their pink ribbons and are kicking ass wherever they go.

I couldn't even make it through a day of transferring phone calls, let alone scale a mountain. I didn't beat cancer and triumph over chemo treatments. In fact, I ran as fast as I could in the opposite direction.

I had done the most drastic thing one could do to *avoid* what cancer patients like Heather were going through. And now I was tired? Poor baby, right?

The shame was exhausting. Finally, I did what I needed to do. New boobs, new body, new life. I needed to go.

I'VE MADE A HUGE LITTLE MISTAKE

My feet are relatively close in size, and besides one of my legs being longer than the other, I am pretty even. My new breasts are pretty close to perfect, but they have minor differences.

So when I had my mastectomy and Dr. Gemignani removed the EXACT same amount of breast tissue from both sides of my body, I took for granted that things would remain pretty even. But when my body healed, my breasts were slightly different. No matter how many experts I paid to make them perfect, my body had a different idea. First, the left breast has a slightly pointier shape than the right. Which was originally ignored because we were going to build a nipple on that mini mountain, but so far I haven't pulled the nipple trigger. Second, the right breast has a dreaded skin wrinkle. The wrinkle is probably my least favorite.

Still, I healed wonderfully. The scars are minimal, and I look completely perfect in low-cut tops. I never have to wear a bra, and I can wear backless dresses. I have two additional tiny dots for scars under my armpits. In all, I am very lucky.

I try not to notice the boob wrinkle. The wrinkle in my perfect-boob plans. The right side of my chest developed more scar tissue around my implant than my left. I can't say for sure why. Maybe because I am right-handed? It could have to do with a million things: how my muscle was cut during the mastectomy, how my arms healed, because I had a gypsy throw a curse on me.

Whatever it is, it's only noticeable when I flex my right pec muscle. You can see the skin on my pecs curl up and wrinkle slightly. It isn't that big of a deal, but whenever I see it, I get embarrassed. It has almost become an automatic reaction to check if my boob is buckling.

If I'm wearing a bra, it's not noticeable at all, but sometimes I catch it wrinkling up during sex, but I am working to let it go. Allen couldn't care less because he's focused on other body parts anyway. It's something I need to accept like criticism or that weird zit in the middle of my back I can't reach.

There is, actually, one other small problem. "Yeah . . . we probably should have gone larger," Dr. Pusic said as she examined my new chest. During my yearly checkup after my reconstruction surgery, we both weren't happy with my breasts. Something just didn't look right. They weren't the correct shape, and they didn't look the same as when I first had the surgery. My breasts looked slightly rectangular.

Originally, Dr. Pusic recommended I go slightly larger when we first chose the implants a year before, but remember that I fought so hard to pick smaller ones. And now once the dust had settled, we could both clearly see she had been right. Because DUH, SHE IS THE DOCTOR—a highly trained medical professional and an expert in breast reconstruction. She does this all day long. I was just a high-strung girl with a doughnut addiction. Why hadn't I listened to her in the first place? I was on a bit of a bitty-titty power trip.

I campaigned for smaller implants because my worst fear was to have this surgery and walk away with breasts that once again drowned me in cleavage. I had dreamed for years about having small breasts—light, weightless, effortless, and completely in my control. It turns out I have no idea what I am doing.

These new breasts weren't working for me. When I looked in the mirror, my new boobs almost seemed droopy. They sloped down at the sides and looked like they folded into my armpit, like I had some overzealous back fat. Repeat: overzealous back fat. It was in fact due to the small size of my implant. They almost looked boxy and not the round, robust fake boobs I thought I'd ordered. My breasts looked like two little frownie eyes, making my midsection look like that sad-face emoji.

At first I figured that was just the way your body looked after a mastectomy. I didn't love it, but I also didn't know if this was normal and I should just be grateful I was healthy. Maybe I just had to grin and bear it? Finally, at my follow-up with Dr. Pusic, I confessed my feelings, and after one look she said, "Yeah, I'm not happy with it."

Wait, WHAT? I thought I was just doing one of those Classic Caitlin Moves, where I complain about my appearance until someone tells me, "No, you look fine. It's in your imagination!"

Not this time. There was clearly something wrong, and Dr. Pusic confirmed it. I was immediately self-conscious and angry at myself. Why didn't I just listen to her? *Always trust the woman in good shoes.*

Dr. Pusic explained: When I first had the implant-exchange surgery, I was pleased with the size because my chest was in fact larger at the time. My chest was swollen from the mastectomy and from the implant surgery. My entire body was still puffy while it was recovering. So all of the decisions I made would have been accurate if my body had stayed that bloated. That was why she encouraged me to go larger. I should have listened to her because she is a doctor and I am just a girl who doesn't check her voice mails.

She also explained that as the swelling went down and the implants settled, they would fill the empty space created when they removed my tissue during the mastectomy, something I wasn't even aware of. I am sure she said something very smart and helpful during that time, but I was on my breast high horse and didn't hear. I was determined never to have large breasts again! As long as my breasts were smaller, I thought I'd be okay. But it turns out I don't like my chest to look like a crying cartoon. I do care.

We scheduled another surgery. This was a hard pill to swallow. I was no longer making an exciting change in my life and future and preventing cancer. This surgery was because I made a big little mistake. Technically, two of them. This was embarrassing, I had to eat 450 ccs of humble pie.

I had to ask family help me once again. There were no cameras around this time. I didn't feel heroic or *Glamorous.* I just felt dumb. From now on, I swore to myself, I'll always take my doctor's advice and keep my DIY eyes on making my new coffee table.

This time, not only did we exchange my implants for ones slightly larger, but Dr. Pusic also used a little of my own fat from my waist and hips and injected it into my chest to add a softer look. I used fat grafting to even out the shape of my new breasts. It gave me a smoother appearance and softened the line between my natural tissue and the new implants. There is a risk that any fat grafted to a new body part might not take and further adjustments might need to be made. As you know, I had worked very hard at self-soothing with food, so they had plenty of material to work with. I have to thank all of the delicious doughnuts and cakes and candies that offered their full support. I don't think this is great for every person, but I enjoyed it.

During my first surgery, I was a noble fighter because the overall goal was avoiding breast cancer. However, now, the reconstruction surgery was purely cosmetic, and I felt the mental shift from "fighting for my life" to "fighting for my sad boobs!" Not as noble, but just as easy to become obsessive and driven to comparisons: *Are mine better or worse than hers?* I used to scoff at my aunt who was a big fan of liposuction and plastic surgery until I did it myself. Having the control of your body to change it is a powerful feeling that is hard to let go of. From now on, I will save my scoffing for celebrities who pretend they were born with thirteen-inch waists and forty-five-inch hips.

Certain celebrities are all over Snapchat and Instagram raving about belly trainers and shapers that are basically modern-day corsets. I wore the same thing when I needed to use liposuction to remove fat from one part of my body to place it in my breasts to adjust their shape. Since the fat was removed from my stomach—thank the good gods above—I had to wear an identical garment as seen by the hottest celebs to help my body and skin readjust. The garment is used to help remove excess fluid from your body and develop your new shape.

And I don't want to throw too much shade, but it's not just boobs they're augmenting—some famous behinds appear to have the impossible shapes that are now promoted in the media. And they can do whatever they want with their bodies. I just want to make sure my little sister doesn't judge herself for not achieving the same results with a million squats. Microscopic waists and large butts that are not natural but possible with plastic surgery and patience. Now that I've done it myself, I can spot the celebs who've done it from a mile away from my TV screen. SHADE.

I cracked the case, just like a real spy! A spy who just had liposuction. I have never been more proud. (And I have never been more nervous about getting sued.) Plus, the surgery once again went well, and I am very happy with the results. My breasts are circular and full, and I now have some cleavage. And my boobs are still on the small side— they just look like full, happy, normal breasts. And I love them. *Finally.*

PREGNANT PLANNED PRESSURE

Before the surgeries, I was rushing Allen to have kids because as soon as I met Allen, I was ready to have all of his kids. I just wanted everything all at once, like the addict I am. Allen wasn't ready to be a father at twenty-two, twenty-five, or twenty-eight, even though I kept asking by playfully joking followed by sobbing during dinner.

Even when I was between temp jobs, when we had absolutely zero money and limited health insurance, when we were first dating, I wanted to have a baby. I have always wanted to have children. When I was a kid, I would pretend to be a mother exhausted with demanding children and household chores. I started babysitting at nine years old and have nannied in between office jobs. I've cleaned more spit-up, poop, and melted Popsicle than I can count.

Still not sure when we will have our babies, but just in case, I have designed a vintage, abstract-autumnal, and Swedish-inspired baby crib. I guess you could say I'm excited: I've already found the perfect onesie in seafoam to match the ocean-blue cable-knit blanket I've commissioned my mom to start making.

I think about what I will tell my children about my mastectomy and breasts. For my girls and boys, I will say the same thing: Mommy had a surgery that will keep her happy and healthy until we are all very old. She's not going anywhere. Some people have blue eyes, and some kids have brown eyes. Mommy was born with boobies that needed a little help. Mommy's doctors made sure she would live a safe and healthy life. Bodies change and that's okay. To my young children I will say my boobies are filled with sparkles and the reason I have scars and no nipples is because the doctor had to seal them up tight so the magic wouldn't spill out. One day my boobies might need to be refilled with applesauce, magic powder, or cocaine—whatever they are into.

I will say that my boobs control Elmo, and if they don't behave, I will give them a squeeze and he will not come back to the TV until they behave. The lies are endless.

I will tell them that everybody is different. Some have white hair and brown lips and soft hands and pointy chins. And we are all just trying to figure it out. I will tell them that they can be brave, and change is okay.

To my teenage daughters I will say, boobs don't matter, all men are gross, and who cares what other kids think? Appreciate it while you have them and delete the naked pictures off your cell phone, because they are never safe. Only French women look good topless.

To my boys I will say breasts are special and don't take them for granted, and also don't touch them. And if you want fake breasts at some point, we can put them under your pectoral muscles too. We are all just on this earth together wanting love, happiness, and free refills.

It might scare my children, but I hope that growing up with a mom who looks like this is just a way of life. And it is something that makes them feel comfortable with other people's bodies and the ways their own bodies look. I will be a mommy with a different body.

Maybe it won't be special at all. Maybe it will just be another thing that they are sick of. They'll be tired of talking about it over dinner and sick of strangers coming up to Mommy, sharing way too much personal information.

I can do my best to educate them and show them the ways we are all different and be as kind and open to them as I possibly can, but they might turn out to be assholes. You never know. Even Mussolini had a mom.

I want to be perfect, but I am pretty sure I will make a lot of mistakes and send my kids running to their therapists with woes of how Mom wouldn't shut up about her health. So Allen and I created a savings account for their future appointments.

OH, SHIT. I FORGOT ABOUT MY OVARIES

At some point, I will have to come to terms with my ovaries and deal with the fact that I also have a high risk of ovarian cancer. That's for another time. Classic Caitlin—I want to hide with the covers over my head while Googling the worst-case scenario.

With my new worry-free boobies, I am happily living without the fear of breast cancer, but it's not like I'm in the clear, cancer-wise. Both BRCA1 and BRCA2 carriers have a higher risk of ovarian cancer than the average women. BRCA1 carriers have a 36–63 percent risk, and BRCA2 carriers have a 10–27 percent risk.[1] Ovarian cancer risk is alarming because ovarian cancer is much harder to detect, and some of the early warning signs are mistaken for other less-threatening conditions. According to the book *Confronting Hereditary Breast and Ovarian Cancer*, by Sue Friedman, DVM, Rebecca Sutphen, MD, and Kathy Steligo, these symptoms are as follows:

- bloating
- pelvic or abdominal pain
- difficulty eating or feeling full quickly
- change in urinary urgency or frequency
- fatigue
- indigestion
- back pain
- pain during intercourse
- constipation
- menstrual irregularities

"Symptoms are particularly significant if they're new, occur every other day or more frequently, and last more than two weeks," they explain. That is why most doctors recommend, after I finish having children, I also have a preventative surgery and remove my ovaries or fallopian tubes. That would mean I would go into early menopause and would probably be on supplemental hormones. Woof. No fun.

The book also says: Removing the breasts and/or ovaries of a healthy woman has implications for fertility and body image. When performed in young women, oophorectomy causes immediate menopause, which can lead to weight gain, an increased risk of cardiovascular diseases, bone loss, and sexual problems."

I don't really want to have an oophorectomy, but I also don't want to get ovarian cancer. So I am currently looking into clinical trials, medication, blood tests, and witch-doctor spells that will help me avoid ovarian cancer and taking out my ovaries before I'm ready.

Until then, it was recommended I go about twice a year for transvaginal ultrasounds and pelvic exams. I'm due for another appointment, and I will totally go. I swear I will, soon, so soon, after I rewatch each season of *Lost*.

I'm banking on medical researchers to keep me from removing my ovaries. If it's medically necessary, once I am finished having babies, I will do whatever is advised by my team of doctors.

Meanwhile, there are my babies to think of. Genetic testing on embryos is a hot topic in the BRCA community. (Turns out, it's not all about nipple stickers.) During this process, doctors artificially inseminate eggs and perform a DNA test to see if they have the BRCA genetic mutation. Doctors will discard the ones that are BRCA positive and supply the mother with only the eggs without the mutation.

I have mixed feelings about embryo genetic testing (preimplantation genetic diagnosis [PGD]), and at the moment I'm not comfortable with the idea. I have had friends tell me it is the solution to end BRCA and others tell me they don't "want to play God." Then again, having this option offers me a great opportunity to avoid my typical panic. I understand both sides, and I am holding firm in my decision to make no decision for now.

I'm going to vaccinate my kids like crazy—don't get shit twisted—but I can't decide if testing my embryos is going too far. When the time is right, I will make another appointment with a genetic counselor to go over all my questions.

Plus, supersmart Anne Marie McCarthy, PhD, instructor of medicine at Harvard Medical School and assistant in epidemiology at Massachusetts General Hospital, reminds me that medical science is always changing. "You are assuming that the conditions today will be the same 30 years from now when this will matter for a child," she said. "As a scientist, I think it's a terrible act of pessimism to select against BRCA or any other genetic condition in an embryo, because you are assuming we won't make any significant progress in helping BRCA carriers in the next 30 years."

Dr. Susan Domcheck, executive director and professor of oncology at the Basser Center for BRCA, whose research on heredity ovarian cancer is wildly revered, also explains she is "always careful about how I talk about PGD. For a lot of women this feels like the right thing to do. It is technology that is available and everyone needs to make their own choice."

SO much to think about, so much worry, so many distractions I can choose to not think about any of it! Meditating on a decision has never been something I've been *great at*. I'm trying to go slowly into this decision. And since it wasn't suggested I have the surgery until I'm forty, I have plenty of time to download a few meditation apps.

MONEY MATTERS

Unfortunately, money matters and it royally sucks. The surgery was covered by insurance and was considered preventative surgery. I was happy because my life would be saved! My insurance company was happy because I was saving them money. The surgeries were cheaper than if I were to develop breast cancer and had to undergo treatments, so they were more than happy to prevent cancer in the process. For the surgeries I had to meet my insurance deductible and then pay my coinsurance for my hospital procedures. They were a fraction of the actual cost of surgery. I did end up paying a little more for extra medication given to me to help with nausea after anesthesia and surgery. Still, there was a hefty bill that I had to pay.

I worked out a plan with the hospital to break down the bill into increments. Even my final surgery, the one that was unexpected, was covered by insurance under the umbrella of reconstruction.

All hospitals have a financial and billing department that is usually willing to work with you on your bills. Get to know them and become friends. Cheryl, in billing, understood this surgery was a large financial burden and went over the systems in place the hospital had to help me with my bill. I found that when I was honest and asked for assistance, they were more than willing to work with me. I think the worst thing to do is to ignore the bills and let them pile up. It just causes Cheryl and me more anxiety than either of us wants.

After surgery I did buy medical bras and silicone nipples and other materials from my hospital, and all of it was covered by insurance. Anything that you might need like specific handmade nipples or organic cotton mastectomy bras might be able to be reimbursed by your insurance. Keep all of the receipts, and then start a claim to see if you can get a little money back. Why not?

You can also save money by putting your gym membership on hold because of a medical condition. Give them a note from your doctor, and it's a free pass out of gym class. Allen and I also cut costs by dropping cable, cooking meals at home more, and asking friends and family to bring us meals instead of candy and flowers. But sometimes we just need to order a pizza, no matter how well we budget, so we do.

CAUTION, CAITLIN: BOOBIES ON BOARD

New boobs, who dis?

Now I actually have the most perfect breasts in the world. I know because it took a team to make them. They don't require a bra or any fancy apparatus. They are cancer free and healthy and all mine! I protect my new breasts like they are two freshly baked pies at risk of being smashed at any moment.

This girl will never say no to a vacation. We were invited to go to Disney World in Orlando for a wedding and family visit. I love Disney. I love the theater majors dressed as Goofy and the plethora of Coke products. I was about nine months after my final surgery, and I was ready to have fun.

My eight-year-old nephew, Cal, loves roller coasters and I consider myself a Fun Aunt, but I had to sit them all out. I am also scared of roller coasters, and I refused to risk any activity that would put any pressure on my chest. So my surgery was a perfect excuse to sit at the bottom of the rides and shop at the Disney Store.

I still want to participate in all the fun activities of life, but I am way more cautious than I was before. Before I was always secretly hoping my big boobs would be cut off in some dramatic explosion in a sword factory. Which would give me an excuse to have a smaller chest. Now I wasn't even going to risk getting too close to a Pirates of the Caribbean display.

I was told by doctors I have to be vigilant in hot showers because it is still very difficult for me to tell temperature while my nerves are still growing back. I will never have the same feeling in my chest as I did before the surgery. I love a good scalding shower, but now I try to keep it a little more under control. I was told not to lean over stoves when cooking or hang over anything sharp because I could be punctured and not notice the impact because I am still numb.

I hate most bras without underwire. They just don't feel as sexy or fun to me; it's the wire that makes it. So, I decided I'd buy overpriced hot-pink underwire bras and then cut out the wire, to keep the glam but lose the danger! Because I CHOOSE ME. If I want to look like a French prostitute from 1957 under my sweatshirt, I have and I will. I'm never not feeling myself up. I'm hypersensitive to any change in my breasts. I am always checking to see if any feeling is coming back or how my scars look. I'm not making excuses for my own paranoia, but it's a good thing I'm obsessed with myself.

I landed a part in a sketch for a comedy Web series! I played a mother carrying her stroller upstairs and struggling. I shook that stroller with all my might and made the director laugh, which was a total rush. I didn't care how many takes we did because I was cast in a three-minute comedy video and I was going for it!

That night I got home and noticed I had huge bruises on my thighs and arms. My left breast looked a little puffy. I didn't realize I had been shaking and throwing the stroller so strongly against my body, but I had the welts to prove it. Since I still have very little feeling in my breasts, I was oblivious to the damage I was happily causing. I immediately called my doctor and her team of nurses. They asked me to come in for the next available appointment, just to be safe. My breasts were examined for discoloration, pockets of fluid, or any irregularity that would cause concern. Luckily, I had only bruises. We were all relieved, and I was sent home and told to ice my chest. If I hadn't made an appointment, I would have panicked all weekend and possibly written another book, "My Puffy Left Breast."

Now all my medical notes include the humbling phrase, "PT states she is a comedian . . ." Clearly, they had their reservations.

I would do that video again in a heartbeat! But next time I will go right to the doctor's office and wait in the waiting room for the bruises to show up. I'm also comforted knowing that it would be awfully hard to actually "break" an implant.

Since surgery, I have felt some nerves starting to grow back, but they feel like nerves attached to my skin and the sensation doesn't go very deep. When I press on my breast, it feels almost identical to when I press on my forearm. Pressing down, I am aware that I am touching my skin, but the feeling is quite shallow. The breast feels similar to my forearm in that I feel the thin muscle on my arm, and then it's stopped abruptly by bone. My current breasts feel that way. They feel like pressing on tissue and muscle, not fake at all, but there is no feeling inside my new breasts because of my implants.

I love these boobs. This is what I wanted all along, smaller boobs that still feel sexy and feminine. (Now I'm the type of girl who can confidently check out her reflection while she walks by a bank.) But I know I won't be floating on this pink cloud forever. My body can and will probably change. Body image has never been easy for me, and there will be moments when I will hate what I see in the mirror. Like last week, when I had the darkest, longest hair coming out of my feminine chin! Ideally, as I age I will be more loving and accepting of my changing body and goatee. And I get to do all of that without worrying about getting breast cancer.

There is a weight lifted—literally. I can now scrutinize my body because of superficial reasons brought on by society rather than the gargantuan burden that was my birth-given bust. Before there was this added element that they would kill me one day or that breast cancer was looming over me, waiting until I was really happy and then ready to strike while I was on an all-inclusive European river cruise.

Now I can just be a normal, insecure, stressed-out woman who is having trouble getting her shirt off in a dressing room. I feel calmer about my future because I know I gave myself my best shot.

I would always love to have Jessica Alba arms and a Kelly Ripa stomach, but at least I'm happy with my chest. Now I can spend time worrying about when I should get Botox and if my cuticles are healthy.

The fat grafting has left a softer, suppler upper breast that when you press on it feels just like a real boob. Let's just call one boob Latkes and one boob Expired Gym Membership.

I actually liked wearing my surgical bras and compression girdles. The "Spanx on steroids" were a symbol of hope while my body felt like it had just been put through a trash compactor.

My breasts now have the permanent perfect shape on my chest as if I were wearing a pushup bra at all times, my décolletage is smooth and full, and my cleavage is even and appropriate. My boobs are the perfect space apart and look proportional in my chest. They fit my frame and my size and are never in the way. When I have sex, they stand proudly without missing a beat. My underboob is soft and smooth and defies gravity. I bet Angelina's does, too!

GIRL, I GOT YOU

After all I've been through, I want to share what I've learned
with others. I've earned some wisdom here, and it would be
selfish of me not to spread it far and wide. Girl, we got this!
Read on for everything you need to know about boob reconstruction but didn't think to ask:

- Everyone wants to touch a fake boob. It's a fact.
- When you bump into something, you can still
  bruise your boob even though you don't feel
  anything.
- My doctor said to be careful when cooking because some women don't notice when they are
  leaning over and might burn themselves. Fine
  with me. I will order Thai mai fun noodles for the
  rest of my life.
- New boobs itch, and I can't always satisfy the
  scratch. Sometimes it helps to move the implant
  around a bit. Yes, you can do that.
- Your scars will fade and lighten with time, just like
  my fascination with Tamagotchi.

- Fat grafting was like winning the lottery. Take that fat off my hips and put it in my boobs? Enough said.
- You might (you will) become obsessed with other people's plastic surgery. Did you even know people get eyebrow lifts? Now you do!
- You will stare at other people's boobs. I'm staring at yours right now.
- Laser hair removal on your breasts doesn't hurt! (Not that either of us has any rogue hairs on our perfect breasts!)
- Your brain may or may not heal faster than your breasts.
- Immediately after surgery, other people's problems feel stupid. Oh, you didn't get that parking space? . . . Wow.
- You can't pick up puppies for a month or two after surgery. Which is devastating.
- Boys will ask questions about your surgery and are even more stupid than you can imagine, like when NASA asked Sally Ride how many tampons she needed to go to space for a week: "Is one hundred the right number?" Yes, that happened![1]

I'M AN OPEN BOOK (UNTIL YOU HURT MY FEELINGS)

I thought *Screw You Cancer* would be perfect for friends and family to be able to share with women in their lives who were exactly in my position and not sure what they wanted to do with their bodies. It was important to me that the videos were online and free. This was about connecting women with as much information as possible and starting a conversation. I almost fell on the floor when they told us we won an Emmy Award for the series! I know! WHAT?! ME? REALLY? Holy shit! How?

After the last of the *Screw You Cancer* videos aired, I had a Facebook and Twitter chat scheduled with *Glamour* and wanted to connect with more women who might be afraid to ask me questions in person or weren't able to. Since my boobs were all over the Internet anyway, I figured why not post it on my personal Facebook page and see if it could spread awareness to my friends?

I was incredibly honored and thrilled that my story traveled so far. I had women reach out to me from all over the world. Friends of friends linked my story and would share any information I provided. I didn't mind sharing at all. I just kept thinking of that nervous girl who feels like she is all alone (that was me). I expected a few comments from people who had no idea what the surgery was or felt strongly that apricot seeds cure cancer. I was fine with that.

Well, not exactly fine . . . I did lose my shit a little after I got a mean comment from some guy I went to high school with. I was expecting criticism, and there was one comment that really hit me hard: Theo wrote something like "What an abomination. It's like slapping God in the face." I am paraphrasing slightly because I deleted the comment from my wall and blocked him quickly after. But he did use all of those words. Why couldn't he just quietly stalk me on Facebook? That's what God would have wanted. But Theo is entitled to his opinion. His stupid, stupid opinion.

I am not friends with Theo in real life, but I am thrilled to know that he's back on speaking terms with God and he can give me the dish. I should ask him more questions since he and God are so close. Will I ever win the lottery? Why is that mole on my hip shaped like a heart? Where does God stand on the constant cross-breeding of dogs? And is THAT how you slap God in the face? Was his face that close to my breasts this whole time?

I had no idea. I must be pretty important. Thank you, Theo, for letting me know that my freedom of choice is something that God hates. Now that you have all the answers, maybe you can finally get a job and move out of your parents' shed? Was that a low blow? Can you ask God for me? This is all such new cool stuff.

Before I had a chance to block him, I was shocked by how many friends and strangers came to my rescue. They went to bat for me, explaining what I did was my own personal choice. They outcommented him until there was nothing left for him to say. THEN I blocked him.

When the videos were first released, I was ready for this situation times ten. "How could someone be so extreme?" "She is irrational!" "Her period made her do it!" I was ready to have to defend my decision to many insane, angry hordes of strangers because I was opening myself up and sharing this personal experience.

I was nervous people thought I wasn't being respectful to women who have had cancer and that my smiling face was annoying or rude. I was ready to join them and started to judge myself. What was I doing? Why would anyone care about my story since I am really a nobody?

Instead, we got two negative comments and hundreds of messages filled with encouragement, joy, and compassion. I was shocked by the support and love freely given by complete strangers. They would watch my entire series and asked great questions. Women wanted updates on my recovery and even prayed for me. It was incredibly humbling. These women reached out in significant numbers and shared their personal stories with me. Whether it was on the phone, over lunch, or through an e-mail, I learned about their experiences. I sat with one woman before her doctor appointment and helped her talk out her nerves. Something I longed for, to have someone know exactly what I needed to hear, and I was lucky enough to give that to her.

After releasing *Screw You Cancer*, I opened my world to all of these brave women. I was asked to speak in other countries about my experience or meet privately with someone's daughter who just needed to share what she was going through. They helped me more than they know. *Screw You Cancer* helped me come out of hiding. It was remarkable, and I was completely blown away.

Screw You Cancer won a Television Academy Honors (a more specific Emmy Award, I was told), and we went to LA for the honoree award ceremony. I was so flipping excited! I took my sister as my date and had my hair and makeup done, and I felt incredible. I looked like I should be walking the red carpet for the CMT Awards, but hey—it was my first red carpet. I wanted my hair to be as big as my excitement.

The series also won an Ellie Award from the American Society of Magazine Editors, and when they announced my name, I burst into tears. This little series that was so special to me and my family was receiving all kinds of recognition, and it was totally shocking.

Everything we had set out to do was achieved and then some. I want to be the friend they can call on when they are fighting their feelings. I can't cure cancer and I am not a celebrity who can pay for cancer-prevention funding, but I can share my story. And we all know I can't keep my mouth shut, so it's basically my destiny. I can talk their ears off and am happy to listen to everything they are going through. It's the most powerful thing I can do.

FAMILY MATTERS

Time passed, as it does. Between my mastectomy and my reconstruction surgery, Allen's father passed away. It crept up on us as we were doing our best to juggle everything. As a result, he assumed full responsibility for his grandmother, who had just moved into a nursing home in Baltimore, a four-hour drive away. Now our kitchen table that was already full of my medical documents was quickly joined by hers. We had to figure out how to sell his grandmother's house, get power of attorney, and manage her care. So we did the most adult thing we could at the time: We asked for help.

Allen didn't have an easy relationship with his father, and now his father was gone. We were thrown into a serious space. We were in hospitals and going to doctor appointments all over again. We were newly married and facing another huge journey.

Allen's mother would call and send over care packages, all while she was dealing with her own grief. She was very proud and told all of the teachers she worked with at her school about my story. She always thought I was braver than she was, but she had beaten cancer numerous times, so I am not sure how that added up in her mind.

Allen's mom was horrible at being modest about her children. She never learned how and didn't really care to. She would proudly show off pictures of Allen and me to her friends at work and tell everyone that we were the coolest and smartest people in New York City. In that way, she reminded me of my family whom I had lost. They took every chance to brag about how proud they were of our accomplishments. She was pushy and often hard to be around, but she loved us more than anything in the world.

Now Allen had a healing wife, bossy dog, full responsibility of his grandmother, and just lost his father. Fear of breast cancer was replaced by a new set of anxieties. Times had changed. It was a new world. Now we were on the giving end in our family, and it felt good, and right, even though it was hard.

It also got me thinking about how my mastectomy was a gift I could give my father. Weirdest gift to date, but now he never has to worry that he will lose me to breast cancer. He was raised with heaps of Jewish guilt, and that was before he learned I got the BRCA mutation from his genes. I have no idea how my dad managed, because I feel bad if I wake my dog up from a nap.

My father never asked me to have the surgery or pressured or even suggested I make that decision. He just wanted me to be informed and to stop canceling my doctor appointments. But not waiting to have the surgery meant he had a few bonus years of relief. This surgery practically guaranteed he won't have to relive any of those tragic moments. I'm terrible at birthday gifts. I've given him white-chocolate golf balls every single year, so hopefully this mastectomy makes up for a few. My dad has been there protecting me since I came into this world, and now this is one less threat he has to worry about. I still have to text him when I'm walking home by myself at night—obviously, that's mandatory. But this time, I gave him something to help him sleep at night, too. Is this what being a grown-up feels like?

ME AS OF FIVE MINUTES AGO

The struggle is *still* real. I didn't suddenly have total peace. Go figure! One night Allen said casually that he sometimes misses my boobs because he loved them. That broke my heart. He would never experience them again. Did he regret my having the surgery this whole time? Is he going to be unsatisfied for the rest of our marriage?

I had a solid week when I regretted the entire surgery and couldn't stop replaying the conversation over in my head. Allen didn't mean to make me feel that way and wasn't expecting this response. He explained, "If you cut off your arm, I would still say, 'Oh, remember when you had an arm?'" He explained that the memories don't just evaporate, which I guess is true, but I had banked on amnesia. I tried to move past my new worries and focus on the fact that I loved my decision and Allen was just being honest about his experience.

The next week we received my original medical photos from my first visit with Dr. Pusic. They were pictures of my old breasts in all their glory. Allen took one look and said, "Oh, God, I forgot how BIG they were. *Those were a pain*. I like these ones much better." Like he was picking between pumpkin pie and apple pie. I almost cried with joy. "Those were so hard on your back," he added. He was brought back to reality quickly, and we could finally let go of those rose-colored memories.

I told him how worried it made me when he missed my breasts, and now he regularly tells me I made the right decision. This guy knows what he's doing. My boobs aren't for anyone's pleasure but mine and—when I'm up for it—my husband's. I'm finally comfortable telling my husband: "No, you need to grab my boobs." It took him a few months because he was worried he would hurt me. Sure, after surgery he would have, but now I'm up for grabs! It doesn't feel like it used to, but it still feels really good. It's a sensory memory (is that a thing, or did I just make that up?) that feels better emotionally than physically. And now if he grabs them and then lets go, they won't drop three feet!

After my third surgery, Allen's cousin Breanna and her fiancé, Curtis, came to visit and stayed with us. They were visiting New York City for the first time and meeting me for the first time. It was only one week after my last implant-exchange surgery. My medication station was still in use, and the house was a mess. Allen's father had just passed away, so he was happy to be around family. I didn't want to be selfish; I wanted to be supportive. So I ignored all my dreadful thoughts about how awful I looked and felt. It was more important for me to ensure Allen was supported by people he loved, because he had been so incredible to me during this entire process. Breanna and Curtis arrived on our doorstep, and it was one of the best parts of my recovery.

I tried my best to be a happy host. I lit a few candles and did the dishes, but I still kept apologizing. This isn't how I usually like to host. Breanna sweetly responded, "We're family. If we can't help each other, who can?" They were ready to be a part of the team. They had a wonderful trip and supplied our home with love and laughter and didn't mind if I had to excuse myself to go rest. She kept reminding me, "This is what family does!"

She's right. I never could have gotten through this without family. I also have never forgotten I was able to have this surgery only because I was sober. If I had kept drinking, I would have washed down the scary idea of a "mastectomy" during Unlimited Sake Mondays. I never would have dealt with my feelings.

Being sober and around other alcoholics in sobriety, everyone is incredibly honest. You have to be to stay sober. Living in the present and sharing our war stories, no rock is left unturned. Harboring and hiding feelings will make sobriety only harder or even impossible. When I put down alcohol, I couldn't hide anymore.

When I was drinking, I didn't have the confidence to put my needs first and was too scared to express them. Because I had practiced this rigorously honest lifestyle for more than a few years, I was able to live that way in the moment. Being sober was the only way I could process these fears and pain and worry. I thought ending drinking would be walking away from a huge part of my world, but it actually opened my eyes to a life greater than I could have imagined. Before I was filled with cliché beliefs, like *When my body is perfect, I will:*

. . . be on time for everything

. . . lounge around all day smoking cigarettes and drinking coffee, but it will look cool and I will never get cancer

. . . maintain a perfect posture while watching the *Price Is Right*

. . . look good in tea-length skirts

. . . be a faster reader

. . . go to IKEA and purchase whatever I want from the showroom floor

. . . invent a car that looks like a bumper car with thick padding around the sides so I will never get injured in a car crash

. . . be friends with celebrities and talk about important things like hospital-patient advocacy and carpools

. . . install a self-cleaning bathroom

. . . invent a walk-in refrigerator that doesn't lock behind you (check if this has already been invented)

. . . enter the Great British Bakeoff and win first prize by making something with raspberry and almond cream, making the judges regret years of eating sad cardboard Oreos

. . . write a series of children books with characters that teach children to reach emotional maturity after reading a few pages

. . . discover my writing is used as an example of strength and hope and great spelling

My body will never actually be perfect, like I might never be able to pick my forever nipples. Which is a relief because now it means I get to see Dr. Pusic whenever

I want. Because the entire reason I even had the surgery in the first place was just a ploy to get closer to her so she would finally tell me where she gets those shoes!

This year I finally gave up my fad-diet fantasies and saw a certified nutritionist. In the flesh. A real human woman who has an actual office, not an avatar who sends you text messages. So far, she is my new lifeline. And like all my doctors, I am still waiting for an invitation to her son's bar mitzvah.

There are nutritional elements I can incorporate in my life to help with cancer prevention, and just now am I able to give them space in my brain. I am no longer hunting for a cure-all diet. This week I am *just* looking for organic fish-oil supplements for my dog.

It took me a mastectomy and two reconstruction surgeries to finally start being kind to my body. Never in a million years did I ever think my breasts would one day lead me to a healthy relationship with food and body acceptance.

PHOTO RESHOOT

The photographer shook her head. "Caity, you *know* that's a stupid face." Ha! And I did! I was having too much fun. I couldn't take myself seriously. My dear friend, and professional photographer, Melissa was taking my photos for my new head shots, after my final surgery. New boobs! New body! Time for new head shots, right? I couldn't wait to get back in front of a camera, with the most honest photographer I know.

I had to keep my shoulders back, raise my chin, and lose the smirk. That's *all* I had to worry about. We didn't have to hide my breasts, hold anything in, or camouflage my body. Blazers were prohibited.

"Let's try another angle. Turn to your left." I was eager to take her suggestions, picturing a tiny Tyra Banks on her shoulder providing feedback. Tiny Tyra never disappoints.

I was having fun. Actual fun. Feeling confident and not apologizing for my body—who was I?! We tried to do some shots without a smile, but I couldn't keep a straight face—never have, never will. I couldn't stop laughing. We tried shirts and different dresses depending on the color or shape

I liked, not based on the threat of cleavage. I finally had my '80s-montage moment!

I, of course, wore Spanx and wanted my arm fat to be hidden—that will never change. But I was confident being straightforward, up close, and every inch of my now perfect chest. There it was again, the lights, the camera, the styling products. This was my victory lap home.

Now I could proudly send my photos to casting directors and agents without fear of being cast as Pregnant Door-to-Door Salesman. And it worked! This year I was cast in a commercial for a cell phone battery and a deodorant commercial. It might not seem like a big deal to someone else, but with each experience I was living my dream. It felt unbelievable to be on a set, in front of a camera, and doing what I love.

Here I am on a more recent shoot, with another great photographer, Alex. Alex takes photos for all the hosts on

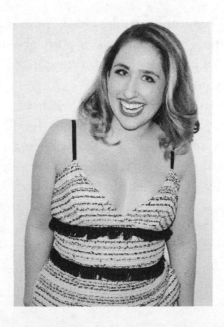

SNL. I KNOW—SO COOL! I tried to act chill, but I just ended up making deeper eye contact.

I had to snap out of it. This was bigger than me and even *SNL.* These photos were to show any girl considering the surgery that she can feel powerful and strong and beautiful after. I wanted to take back the typical postsurgical photos. There are plenty taken in front of a blue wrinkled curtain in the back of the doctor's office, and I wouldn't exactly call them "inspirational."

I know, because before my surgery I wanted to see every iteration of breasts after reconstruction. I just wanted to get as many clues as to how my body would change. I wanted to touch them and feel the heft. Honestly? Who doesn't?

The hardest part was imagining how I would look in dresses and wondering if I would have scars that would show in tank tops or if my underboob would be smooth. So I had a job to do. Give the girls what they want. We shot the photos in his studio, and Alex couldn't have been more excited.

I was stunned at how comfortable I was in my own skin. This was new! I changed tops and dresses and had conversations topless. There are no nipples, so there's nothing to hide. I would have been mortified if any professional photographer saw my melons before. Now I was sipping coffee while picking out the next outfit, without covering up and without a care in the world. Who was I? We focused on hair and makeup and lights and shadows, and the size of my breasts was *never brought up.*

My body isn't perfect, but I love how much it has changed. And I don't think that this surgery will bring total body acceptance for every woman, but I definitely changed.

I still have my hang-ups, as outlined in this entire book, but even those don't feel like the end of the world. It's been a few years, but I am proud of the decisions I have made. Body. Be. Bangin.

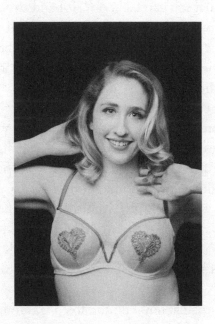

And now, since my body is right where I want it and I am finally feeling like myself again, it's time to blow shit up and make a baby! Allen is into it, or at least I think he's into it. Hopefully, he will be into it, when I tell him, which I will very soon . . . and then we can focus on baby making, and honey, you know I'm gooooood at that.

THE LAST OF MY ADVICE

Hopefully, my experience can be a help to anyone considering a preventive mastectomy. Or maybe my story is just a complicated cautionary tale for anyone considering auditioning for an infomercial?

There's only so much advice I can give you. Every woman should decide what's right for her own body. Whether she's thinking about dieting or avoiding cancer or having surgery to look and feel better, that's a personal choice, and I hope you make the decisions that are right for *you*. My best advice: keep yourself educated, make sure you have a supportive medical team, and never, ever undervalue free snacks.

If you believe you could be BRCA positive or at risk for cancer, after connecting with a doctor or genetic counselor, I would recommend reaching out to a support group and becoming involved in the hereditary cancer community. Connecting with others who are in the same position makes everything easier. Trust me. I know!

Before I say good-bye, here are a few handy checklists for you to use if you ever have your very own breast surgery.

Why reinvent the wheel, right? These will save you the trouble of coming up with your own stupid questions and weird anxieties. You can just use mine and go home early.

Dumbest Questions I Asked the Nurse

- Will it hurt?
- Will my scars be really big?
- What if I get my period in the middle of surgery? Will you hate me?
- Will my boobs look weird?
- How soon after surgery can I have sex?
- Will I pee or poop myself during surgery?
- How will I go to the bathroom after surgery?
- Do you like me, and if so, can we be friends?

Top Fears: One Week Before Surgery

- My boobs will suddenly combust.
- I will change my mind in the middle of surgery and be crying out from a dream.
- This is a huge mistake.
- I won't be able to lift my arms again because something terrible will go wrong during surgery.
- I will love the pain meds.

Top Fears: One Day Before Surgery

- My boobs will suddenly combust.
- It will hurt too much to move and then I will forget how.

- I will miss out on fun things while I am recovering.
- I won't be able to thank Allen enough for all he is doing.
- I will pee myself during surgery.

Top Fears: One Hour Before Surgery

- My boobs will combust.
- I didn't hug my family hard enough.
- I won't fall asleep once they give me the meds.
- I forgot to pee.

Presurgical Advice

- Get an armpit wax. You won't be able to wax or shave for a while. While you're at it, get that bikini wax too.
- Get a gel or semipermanent manicure. While you have an IV in your hand, you can look lovingly on your beautiful cuticles and not stress.
- Buy a lot of perfume and baby wipes. You won't be able to shower until you get the okay from the doctor—and you will get a LOT of visitors who all want to hug you and come superclose.
- Get your hair DID, DONE, DO IT ALL, and invest in good dry shampoo, because like earlier, you won't be able to shower or get your hair done for days and you will hate looking at your oily roots.
- Your boobs won't explode, but you might pee a little.

More Presurgical Advice

- Don't tell your anesthesiologist you are a comedian.
- Not everyone wants to talk about cancer when you want to talk about cancer.
- Be nice to your body: it has done nothing wrong and wants to be friends again.
- You do not need everyone's advice.
- Take some boobie selfies to remember them in future moments of nostalgia.
- People love the word *boobs*. This will never change.
- You may always want to lose nine pounds and may always hate going to the gym.
- You aren't going to die from fear, even though it feels that way.

And never forget: I am here for you if you need anything.

xo,

Caitlin

ACKNOWLEDGMENTS

THANK YOUUUUUUUUUUUUUUUUUUUUUUUUUU UUS!!! I still can't believe I wrote an entire book and that you are still reading it! I couldn't have done this without my tribe of loving mentors, friends, and family members who helped me along the way. I am sure I will forget someone who helped me, like a Hollywood starlet at the end of her acceptance speech. Except this is at the end of a heavily revised book and I am very sober.

Special thanks to my incredible agent, Hannah Gordon, for taking a chance on me and fighting for me from day one. You believed in me from the very start and worked constantly to make sure this book was a reality. You have taken so many of my calls and "OMG" e-mails with grace. I am just so grateful for your hard work and patience.

Thank you to my marvelous editor, Laura Mazer, for being my book mother. Thank you for your wisdom, kindness, brilliant feedback and patience. I adore working with you. Thank you to my hysterical copy editor, Annette Wenda, brilliant project editor, Michael Clark, and proofreader, Suzie Tibor, for your patience and sharp eyes.

Thank you to Mathew Weston and my incredible bad ass publicists, Sharon Kunz and Kathleen Carter Zrelak.

Thank you Rachel Bloom for being extremely generous. Your heart is huge, and I am forever grateful. You really are just a tremendous talent and just the FU%&$#*@ KING BEST! Thank you to my Upright Citizens Brigade community of hysterical friends who made me a funnier, stronger writer. Thank you for reading early copies and for your helpful feedback and ideas. Special thank you to the very funny Nikki Palumbo, Cara Devins, and Gwynna Forgham-Thrift for great feedback like "ARE YOU TAKING A STAB AT PAULA POUNDSTONE?!?!?!!" and for Mike Scollins for that great idea and his continued support from the very start.

Thank you Ariel Elias for your funny feedback, and thank you for reminding me to include a special thank you to the senior citizens at the Steinway Queens Library who sat next to me as I finished this book, specifically Edward and Nick, and the old man who mainly naps.

Thank you Ilana Glazer and Abbi Jacobson for being wonderfully kind friends and supporting me and this book from the beginning. Big thank you to Sara Benincasa for being such a wonderful friend and for talking me through an "I can't finish this book" panic attack.

Thank you Neil Simon, for being my friend and mentor and telling me I was a writer before I knew I could be one.

Thank you Eric Schrier, Kerry Horn, and Elena Raines for your help and great advice. Thank you Eric Silver, Jon Gutierrez, and Lawrence Kern for your comic book guidance. So grateful for Nikki Franjakis for being a brilliant stylist and a kind friend. Thanks to Alex Schaefer and Mindy Tucker for the incredible photos. And thank you to my website designer, Alexandra Fiber.

Thank you to the team of medical experts who helped me fact-check and gave me priceless guidance: Anne Marie McCarthy, PhD; Mary L. Gemignani, MD, MPH, FACS; Susan M. Domchek, MD; Dr. Noa Shemesh; Sharon Bober, PhD; Udi Arad, MD; Payal D. Shah, MD; and Claudine Isaacs, MD.

I am extremely grateful to Andrea Pusic, MD, MHS, FRCSC, for taking the time to help edit my medical chapters and for your continued kindness and for not kicking me out of your office after my sixth visit to "discuss nipples." Thank you to the nurses at Memorial Sloan Kettering Cancer Center. Thank you for your patience and for always being prepared for any puking that might accompany my visit. Thank you to Dr. Sue Friedman and the FORCE community for their support. Thank you to my BRCA sisterhood of survivors, previvors, and brave women. Thank you Basser Center, NYU Langone, NIH, and Cancer.org for your guidance.

Thank you to Angelina Jolie. No, you don't know me, but your honesty and bravery changed my life. Enormous thanks to *Glamour* magazine for allowing me to share my story and to the team of *Screw You Cancer*, Cathryne Czubek, Grant Jones, Michael Klein, Matt Porwoll, Ann Saks, and everyone at CNE and Glamour.com for your hard work and support. Thank you, Megan Angelo, for making it all happen. Thank you, Cindi Leive, for making my dreams come true by supporting my story as you support so many other women.

Adriana and Lauren, thank you for being the most incredible friends and for letting me hold your hands during the entire process.

Thank you to my huge family of cousins, aunts, uncles, grandparents, and in-laws who gave me constant love and support and Edible Arrangements. Thank you to Kenzie for loving me and always being there for every single feeling, thought, or worry I have and being on call to discuss all of it in great detail. I love you so much, and I am here to protect you always. Thank you, Conor, for letting me smother you with love and worry and for being a calm, supportive brother and friend during this entire process. Thank you for telling me I could write this book when I was positive I could not. Thank you to my parents for protecting me and loving me harder than I could even imagine. For my mom for holding my hand through my life, through my surgery, and while writing this book. Thank you, Dad, for believing in me, protecting me, loving me always, and for walking my dog. Thank you, Bubby, for smothering me with love and support. I miss you. Thank you to my Poppy, Iris, and Valia. I hope I made you proud. And thank you, Allen, for being my favorite person. You milked my drains, and then you read every draft of my book. You have spent more hours than I knew were possible loving me. I was only able to do this because you picked me up so many times and brushed me off and told me I was capable and smart enough to finish this book. I am so lucky to be by your side, and I am a better writer and kinder person because of you. Thank you for waking me up from every nap because I consistently sleep through alarms.

I love you all,

Caity

NOTES

Introduction

1. The lifetime risk of breast cancer was 82 percent. Lifetime risks of ovarian cancer were 54 percent for BRCA1 and 23 percent for BRCA2 mutation carriers (https://www.ncbi.nlm.nih.gov/pubmed/14576434). D. Ford et al., "Risks of Cancer in BRCA1-Mutation Carriers. Breast Cancer Linkage Consortium," *Lancet* 343 (March 1994): 692–695; M. C. King et al., "Breast and Ovarian Cancer Risks Due to Inherited Mutations in BRCA1 and BRCA2," *Science* 302 (October 24, 2003): 643–646.

2. Jacques Raphael et al., "The Impact of Angelina Jolie's (AJ) Story on Genetic Referral and Testing at an Academic Cancer Centre," 2014 Breast Cancer Symposium, http://meetinglibrary.asco.org/content/136716-151.

Cancer Is an Emotionless Bitch Who Will Ruin Your Brunch Plans

1. E. Y. Tang et al., "Population-Based Study of Attitudes Toward BRCA Genetic Testing Among Orthodox Jewish Women," *Breast Journal* (November 30, 2016).

2. O. M. Ginsburg et al., "BRCA1 and BRCA2 Families and the Risk of Skin Cancer," *Familial Cancer* 4 (December 2010): 489–493; Bernard Friedenson, "BRCA1 and BRCA2 Pathways and the Risk of Cancers Other than Breast or Ovarian," *Medscape General*

Medicine 7, no. 2 (2005): 60; Jacqueline Mersch et al., "Cancers Associated with BRCA1 and BRCA2 Mutations Other than Breast and Ovarian Cancer," *American Cancer Society* 121 (September 15, 2014); C. R. Ferrone et al., "BRCA Germline Mutations in Jewish Patients with Pancreatic Adenocarcinoma," *Journal of Clinical Oncology* 27 (January 20, 2009): 433–438; E. Castro et al., "Germline BRCA Mutations Are Associated with Higher Risk of Nodal Involvement, Distant Metastasis, and Poor Survival Outcomes in Prostate Cancer," *Journal of Clinical Oncology* 31 (May 10, 2013): 1748–1757. See also http://www.onclive.com/publications /obtn/2013/may-2013/genetic-basis-for-poor-prognosis-in-prostate -cancer-identified#sthash.3jhmMrXq.dpuf.

Google's Land of Horrors

1. J. M. Satagopan et al., "Ovarian Cancer Risk in Ashkenazi Jewish Carriers of BRCA1 and BRCA2 Mutations," *Clinical Cancer Research* 8 (December 2002): 3776–3781.

2. "What to Do If Your Genetic Test Results Are Positive," http://www.breastcancer.org/symptoms/testing/genetic/pos_results.

3. Anne Marie McCarthy and Katrina Armstrong, "The Role of Testing for BRCA1 and BRCA2 Mutations in Cancer Prevention," *JAMA Internal Medicine* 174 (July 2014): 1023–1024.

4. Susan M. Domchek et al., "Association of Risk-Reducing Surgery in BRCA1 or BRCA2 Mutation Carriers with Cancer Risk and Mortality," *JAMA* 304, no. 9 (2010): 967–975.

Oh, Shit. I Forgot About My Ovaries

1. Ibid.

Girl, I Got You

1. Adam Cole, "What Happens When You Get Your Period In Space?," September 17, 2015, http://www.npr.org/sections/health -shots/2015/09/17/441160250/what-happens-when-you-get-your -period-in-space.

ABOUT THE AUTHOR

Caitlin Brodnick is a comedian and public speaker. She performs at Upright Citizens Brigade Theatre New York and has written for Glamour.com and *Huffington Post*. Caitlin created the docuseries *Screw You Cancer* with *Glamour* magazine. The series went on to win a National Magazine Award for Best Video and was awarded a Television Academy Honor (Emmy) in 2013 for using the power of television and video media to bring awareness to important social issues. Caitlin lives in New York City with her husband and bossy dog.